AF444963

BARLEY GRASS JUICE

From the Grass Juice Factor to Modern Scientific Evidence

MICHAEL S DONALDSON, PHD

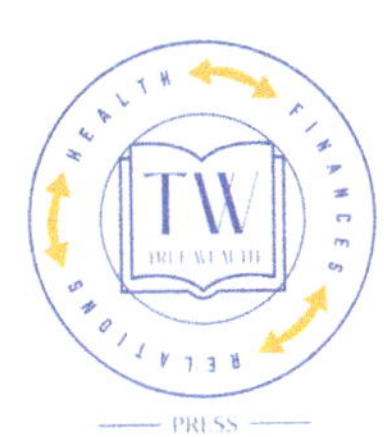

Copyright © 2026 by Michael S Donaldson, PhD

ISBN-13: 979-8-9963582-0-5 (Paperback edition)

ISBN-13: 979-8-9963582-1-2 (Ebook edition)

All rights reserved.

No part of this book may be reproduced in any form or by any electronic or mechanical means, including information storage and retrieval systems, without written permission from the author, except for the use of brief quotations in a book review.

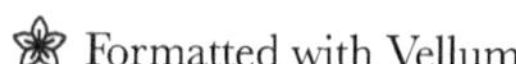 Formatted with Vellum

For George Malkmus, who introduced me to the power of living foods.

Contents

WHY THIS BOOK, AND WHY NOW

Interest in cereal grasses and barley grass juice did not begin recently. Long before "superfoods" entered popular language, careful researchers and clinicians were already documenting the remarkable biological activity of young cereal grasses, effects that no single identified nutrient could account for and that isolated supplements could not replicate.

Two books, in particular, laid important groundwork.

Cereal Grass: Nature's Greatest Gift by Ronald Seibold, published in 1991, presented a comprehensive overview of cereal grass research available at the time. It carefully documented early animal studies, biochemical observations, and practical applications, and it helped preserve scientific work that might otherwise have been lost to obscurity.

Earlier still, *Green Barley Essence: The Ideal 'Fast Food'* by Yoshihide Hagiwara, M.D., published in 1985, introduced many readers to the concept that young barley grass juice was not merely a "green food," but a biologically active substance with unique properties. Dr. Hagiwara's work helped bring attention to barley grass juice as something worthy of serious scientific consideration.

Both of these books were substantial works, each roughly 140–150 pages, and both were excellent for their time. But time matters in science.

The newest of these books is now more than 35 years old. Since their publication, analytical techniques have advanced dramatically. We now understand flavone profiles, antioxidant systems, metabolic signaling pathways, and cellular defense mechanisms in ways that were simply not possible in the 1980s and early 1990s. At the same time, the landscape of chronic disease has shifted profoundly, with diabetes, metabolic syndrome, inflammatory disorders, and depression and chronic fatigue becoming far more prevalent than any of the earlier researchers could have anticipated.

This book exists because that gap has grown too large to ignore.

HOW I CAME TO WRITE IT

I came to this subject not through an interest in supplements, but through a specific scientific problem.

After completing my PhD in chemical engineering at Cornell University in 1998, I joined the research team at Hallelujah Diet, a whole-food health organization with an unusual track record. Their approach centered on raw living foods: fresh vegetable juice, raw fruits and vegetables, and the principle that the biological complexity of living plant foods could not be replaced by isolated nutrients or processed substitutes. What drew me was not the philosophy but the results. People were recovering from chronic diseases using dietary approaches that conventional medicine had not prioritized. The anecdotal evidence was stronger than what I had seen associated with many more heavily funded interventions. Something was working, and I wanted to understand what.

My first research priority was deceptively simple: how do you prove, scientifically, that a food has not been cooked? Every claim about the value of raw living foods rested on the assumption that the product being consumed actually retained its biological vitality. Enzyme testing turned out to be the most sensitive and reliable answer. Enzymes are fragile. They are among the first casualties of heat, oxidation, and rough handling. A food that retains robust enzyme activity has been processed gently enough that its most vulnerable components survived. A food without measurable enzyme activity has not.

That method eventually led me to barley grass juice powder, and to a discovery I did not expect.

Around 2001, a sample of barley grass juice powder arrived at our laboratory. It had been sitting in a corner, unexamined. When I ran it through our enzyme panel and compared the results to every other barley grass product we had tested up to that point, the numbers were striking. Fresh samples of the same product were better still. It outperformed everything we had seen.

That single unexamined sample was how we found the producer who has supplied the highest-quality barley grass juice powder I have encountered in more than 27 years of independent testing work. I will return to that story in detail in Chapter 10, where the testing methodology is laid out fully, and the results of comparative enzyme and chlorophyll analysis across commercially available products are presented directly.

WHAT THIS BOOK IS, AND WHAT IT IS NOT

What you will find here is not a repetition of earlier material, nor an attempt to romanticize cereal grass as a cure-all. Instead, this book brings together what early researchers observed but could not fully explain, what modern laboratory and animal studies now clarify, where limited but important human data fit into the picture, and how all of this translates into practical, realistic use today.

This is not a long book by design. You do not need hundreds of pages to benefit from this research. What you need is clarity: what matters, what does not, and how to apply what we know responsibly.

The research reviewed here was conducted by independent groups in Poland, Egypt, Japan, Nepal, China, Slovakia, and the United States. None of it was commissioned by a supplement manufacturer trying to validate a product. It was driven by the same chain that has always propelled the most trustworthy science: people used barley grass juice, reported results that surprised them, and curious researchers followed the evidence.

If you are looking for exaggerated promises or simplistic answers, this book will disappoint you. If you want a clear, evidence-guided understanding of barley grass juice (what it is, why it works when it does, why it sometimes does not, and how to use it intelligently), this book is meant for you.

At the end of the book, you will find a bibliography for readers who wish to explore the original research further. Science progresses by building on what came before, and this work stands on the shoulders of those who laid the foundation decades ago, including those who understood, long before modern research confirmed it, that what God placed in living plants was worth paying attention to.

This is an update, not a replacement. And it is long overdue.

Michael Donaldson

Ph.D., Chemical Engineering, Cornell University

Chapter 1

LIFE COMES FROM LIFE

Life comes from life. Always. Scientists have never taken any mix of non-living substances and made them into a living organism. Life is always reproduced. Life is never created by us. Life comes from life.

Living beings require living foods to thrive. This is difficult to prove with a single experiment, but the evidence accumulated across more than a century of nutritional research, and confirmed repeatedly in the lives of ordinary people who discovered it through their own suffering, points consistently in the same direction. Whole, living, raw plant foods carry something that processed, cooked, and chemically reduced foods do not. Something that isolated vitamins and mineral supplements cannot replace. Something that the human body recognizes and responds to in ways that no pharmaceutical formulation has yet been able to replicate.

This book is about one expression of that principle found in young barley grass juice and the remarkable science that has accumulated around it. But before we can understand what barley grass juice does and why it matters, we need to understand the larger truth it belongs to. And that truth is best understood not through abstract argument, but through the lives of the people who discovered it.

What Is Special About Living Food?

One of the most measurable differences between living and processed food is enzymatic activity. Enzymes are biological catalysts, molecules that accelerate chemical reactions and make them more efficient than they otherwise would be. Every living cell depends on them. And enzyme activity correlates directly with the vitality of a food: raw, living foods carry robust enzymatic activity, while cooked, processed, and heat-damaged foods carry little or none.

This is not a philosophical claim. It is a measurable, reproducible fact. We can quantify enzyme activity in a food sample using reliable scientific methods, and the measurements consistently show that processing destroys what living plants produce. The more aggressively a food is processed, the less enzymatic life it retains. This principle will become central to everything discussed in Chapters 9 and 10, where we examine what laboratory testing reveals about different barley grass products and why the differences between them matter profoundly.

But enzymes are only the most measurable dimension of what living food carries. The pioneers of raw food nutrition discovered, through their own experience and their patients' recoveries, that something broader and deeper was at work, something that no list of known nutrients could fully account for.

The Laboratory Evidence: Kollath's Landmark Experiment

Before the personal stories, consider the controlled laboratory work of Professor Werner Kollath of Germany, whose experiments before World War II provided one of the earliest and most rigorous demonstrations of the principle that life requires living food.

Werner Kollath fed laboratory animals a purified, highly processed diet containing only potassium phosphate and a small amount of zinc for minerals, and only thiamine as a vitamin. On paper, the diet was nutritionally complete by the standards of his era. And initially, the animals appeared to confirm that. They grew. They developed normally. No obvious clinical signs of disease appeared in their early lives.

But as the animals aged, the picture changed. Dental cavities developed. Constipation set in. The balance of bacteria in the colon shifted in harmful directions. Bone mineral density dropped. And when the animals were examined after death, their internal organs showed damage characteristic of the degenerative diseases seen in aging humans, diseases that should not have been present in animals receiving what appeared to be adequate nutrition.

Professor Kollath then set about identifying what was missing. He tried every vitamin and mineral supplement available. He tried them individually and in combination. None of them restored the animals' health. The only intervention that worked was returning fresh, raw food to the diet. Foods like green leaves, cereal grasses, and raw vegetables. Life, it turned out, could only be restored by life. No chemical inventory of known nutrients was sufficient.

Kollath called the condition he had produced "mesotrophy." He described it as a state of hidden malnutrition in which an organism appears healthy but is being slowly depleted of something essential that no isolated supplement can provide. His work was a quiet but devastating critique of nutritional reductionism decades before that critique became widely accepted.

The Human Evidence: Pioneers Who Discovered What Life Requires

Werner Kollath's laboratory findings were mirrored, independently and repeatedly, in the lives of individuals who turned to raw living foods in desperation and found what conventional medicine had been unable to give them.

Max Bircher-Benner was a young, overworked physician in Switzerland when he was struck with a serious case of jaundice. Unable to eat, he reached for a piece of apple his wife was peeling, and his body accepted it when he could eat nothing else. Days of apples later, he found himself recovering. He applied this discovery hesitatingly to his patients, then with growing confidence, and eventually established a clinic in Zurich where raw, unfired foods were foundational to every treatment. His clinic became internationally known, and his methods influenced nutritional medicine for generations.

Max Gerson was a brilliant young physician suffering from debilitating migraine headaches. Unable to find a medical solution, he used himself as a test case and experimented with dietary change. A milk-based diet made him worse. A fruit-based diet, beginning, like Bircher-Benner, with apples, resolved his migraines entirely. He could verify which foods were acceptable because any dietary misstep brought the headache back. He shared his discovery with a patient who also suffered migraines, and it worked for that individual as well, along with resolving that patient's skin lupus, a benefit Gerson had not anticipated. Albert Schweitzer's wife later used the Gerson approach for tuberculosis. Gerson eventually immigrated to the United States and practiced medicine in New York, using fresh raw foods and vegetable juices as the foundation of his cancer therapy, a story that deserves, and has received, its own book.

Norman Walker recovered from a serious illness by finely grating carrots and pressing out the juice (an act of sheer desperation, I am sure). But this laborious process nonetheless produced results that no other intervention had. His recovery led directly to his invention of the Norwalk juicer and a lifetime of teaching that disease begins in the colon and that fresh vegetable juices provide what processed food cannot. His work introduced thousands of people to the therapeutic power of raw juice.

Ann Wigmore grew up in Lithuania, watching her grandmother treat wounded soldiers in World War I with herbs and natural therapies. After immigrating to the United States as a young adult, she suffered a serious accident that left both legs broken above the ankles. Gangrene developed. Physicians recommended amputation of both limbs. Her father agreed. Ann remembered her grandmother's methods, refused the surgery, and chose a different path — sitting in sunshine, eating grass from the lawn, consuming the flowers her uncle brought her. She recovered completely. The experience shaped the rest of her life. She devoted herself to understanding the healing properties of grasses, eventually settling on wheatgrass as the most practical and potent option for people to grow and juice at home. She treated many people holistically using fresh wheatgrass juice and raw salads as the physical foundation of recovery. Her work became one of the most influential threads in the modern raw food movement.

Reverend George Malkmus was at the height of his pastoral ministry at the age of 42 when he received a diagnosis of colon cancer. His mother had recently died of colon cancer after following standard medical treatment, and that outcome shaped his response to his own diagnosis. Rather than following the same path, he sought counsel from evangelist Brother Lester Roloff, who directed him toward a raw food diet, grounded in the dietary principles described in Genesis 1:29, and large quantities of fresh carrot juice. Within a year, the tumor was gone, along with the other physical ailments that had accumulated from following a conventional diet for a lifetime.

Malkmus was not a scientist, and he would have been the first to acknowledge it. His gift was different: he could reach people. He understood, from his own dramatic recovery, that something in living food did what medicine had not, and he carried that message with extraordinary energy into churches, communities, and living rooms across America. His explanations of the science were not always precise (the mechanisms behind his recovery were not something he could fully account for), but the results he and the people around him experienced were real. Thousands of people who followed his dietary approach and reported meaningful improvements in their health were not imagining things. The science reviewed in this book is, among other things, a belated attempt to explain what those people were experiencing and why.

What Malkmus contributed was not a research program but a movement, a widespread, sustained demonstration that living foods could produce results that conventional approaches had not. That kind of evidence, however imprecise in its framing, is what eventually draws scientific attention. Researchers follow results. Malkmus generated them in abundance, and that is what attracted me to Hallelujah Acres in the first place.

A Pattern That Cannot Be Ignored

These are not isolated anecdotes. They are a pattern, repeated across different countries, eras, medical conditions, and individuals who arrived at the same discovery through entirely separate paths.

Professor Kollath could only reverse the hidden malnutrition in his laboratory animals with raw vegetables. Ann Wigmore restored her legs and her health with raw grasses. Norman Walker recovered from illness with fresh carrot juice. Max Gerson resolved migraines and helped others overcome tuberculosis and cancer using raw foods and vegetable juices. Max Bircher-Benner recovered from jaundice with raw fruit and built a clinic on that foundation. George Malkmus recovered from colon cancer with a raw food diet and fresh juice, and spent the rest of his life sharing what he had found.

The specific foods differed. The conditions differed. The individuals differed. What did not differ was the direction of the evidence. Living food restored what processed food could not maintain and what isolated supplements could not repair.

This pattern has continued long past these pioneers. Countless individuals have followed similar paths, facing serious health challenges, turning to living foods when conventional medicine offered limited options, and finding their way back to health. Their stories are less famous but no less real, and a few of them will be shared in the success stories chapter at the end of this book.

What began with a few determined individuals discovering what God had placed in living plants from the beginning has become a worldwide movement and a body of scientific inquiry that continues to grow. The impetus for researching barley grass juice powder globally has always been the same: people used it, reported results, and curious scientists followed the evidence. That chain, from human experience to laboratory investigation, runs through every chapter of this book.

What This Means for Everything That Follows

Life comes from life. It is not a slogan. It is a biological reality, demonstrated in controlled laboratory experiments, confirmed in the recoveries of people who should not have recovered, and now being mapped at the molecular level by researchers on every inhabited continent.

The chapters that follow examine what modern science has discovered about one specific expression of this principle: young barley grass juice. What it contains. What it does in biological systems. Why its form matters profoundly. And what nearly a century of research, from the earliest animal experiments to the most recent cell culture and molecular studies, reveals about why this ancient plant, harvested at precisely the right moment and processed with sufficient care, continues to produce effects that no isolated supplement has been able to replicate.

The answer, as you will see, was always in the design. And the design was always in the life.

Chapter 2

THE GRASS JUICE FACTOR: A DISCOVERY AHEAD OF ITS TIME

During the 1930s and 1940s, nutritional science was undergoing a profound shift. Researchers had recently identified vitamins A, B, C, D, and E, and there was growing optimism that human health could be explained largely through the discovery of isolated micronutrients. If scientists could simply identify every essential compound, synthesize it reliably, and deliver it in a pill or a powder, the problem of human nutrition might be solved once and for all.

As the previous chapter made clear, this pursuit proved far more complicated than anyone anticipated. Life comes from life, and the reductionist dream of replacing whole food with a collection of isolated chemicals kept running into the same stubborn obstacle: living systems did not respond to chemical inventories the way researchers hoped. Something kept getting left out. Something in whole, living food, something that no one could yet name or isolate, kept making the difference between thriving and merely surviving.

The story of the grass juice factor is one of the clearest early demonstrations of that reality.

A Farmer's Observation Becomes a Scientific Question

The thread begins not in a university laboratory but in a field. In the late 1920s, Charles Schnabel, an agricultural chemist with a practical problem, was looking for a way to improve the health and productivity of his laying hens during the winter months. Chickens in winter are notoriously poor layers. Reduced sunlight, cold temperatures, and limited access to fresh green forage all conspire to suppress egg production. Schnabel tried various interventions, as any farmer would, before hitting on something unexpected.

When he added young cereal grasses to the chickens' diet, specifically grasses harvested while still in their early, rapidly growing stage, the results were striking. Winter egg laying in his hens increased from 38% to 94%. That is not a marginal improvement. It is a transformation, and it was reproducible. Other green vegetables did not produce the same effect. Alfalfa did not produce it. Something specific to young cereal grasses, such as barley, wheat, rye, and oats, was responsible.

Schnabel was not a man to leave an observation unexplained. He began documenting his findings systematically and eventually brought his work to the attention of the broader scientific community. What had begun as a practical farming observation became a genuine scientific question: what was in young cereal grass that produced effects no other green food could replicate?

The University Laboratory Takes Over

It was that question that drew Dr. George Kohler and his colleagues at the University of Wisconsin into the investigation during the 1930s. Kohler was a rigorous researcher working in a well-equipped laboratory, and he approached the grass juice factor with the tools and methods of his era: controlled animal experiments, careful measurement of biological outcomes, and systematic comparison of different dietary interventions.

What he found was remarkable and, at the time, difficult to explain.

Young barley grass juice increased fertility in laboratory animals, specifically by inducing ovulation in females that had not been cycling normally. This was not a subtle hormonal nudge. It was a measurable restoration of reproductive function, the kind of effect that suggested the juice was interacting with fundamental biological processes rather than simply providing calories or basic micronutrients.

Dairy cows fed young grasses saw significant increases in milk production. But the more intriguing finding came from what happened when that milk was consumed by other animals. Guinea pigs sustained on milk from cows that had been grazing on young grasses thrived. Guinea pigs sustained on winter milk, from cows fed standard winter rations without access to fresh young grass, did not fare nearly as well. The factor, whatever it was, was passing from the grass to the cow and from the cow into her milk, where it remained active enough to support the health of animals downstream in the food chain.

The implications extended even further. Infants of nursing women who consumed milk from grass-fed cows developed more rapidly than infants whose mothers drank milk from cows on winter rations. The grass juice factor was not merely sustaining laboratory animals under controlled conditions. It appeared to travel through multiple biological systems — plant to cow, cow to milk, milk to nursing mother, mother to infant — retaining its activity at each transfer. That kind of biological persistence pointed to something genuinely fundamental rather than a nutritional curiosity.

The Search for What It Was

With results this consistent and this significant, the obvious next step was identification. If something in young cereal grass was producing these effects, what was it? Could it be isolated, characterized, and eventually synthesized or concentrated?

Researchers tried. They tried systematically and persistently for decades, ruling out candidate after candidate with the methodical patience that serious science requires. Liver extracts were tested — no match. Whole milk was examined — insufficient. Wheat germ, brewer's yeast, vitamins K, A, D, E, C, B1, B2, B3, B6, folic acid,

B12, inositol, iron, copper, manganese, and zinc were all investigated as potential explanations, either alone or in combination. None of them replicated the effects of young cereal grass juice. Chlorophyll, the most obvious candidate given the juice's green color, was tested and ruled out as the primary factor, though researchers noted that it carried its own beneficial properties.

The factor was essential for the good health of guinea pigs in ways that no known nutrient could replace. It showed up in barley, wheat, rye, and oats, in young white clover, peas, and cabbage to a lesser degree, but the highest concentrations were consistently found in the cereal grasses, and within that group, young barley grass juice produced the strongest and most reliable effects.

Unable to isolate the responsible compound, or compounds, researchers gave the observed activity a descriptive name: the grass juice factor. It was not a name born of ignorance. It was a placeholder, chosen carefully by scientists who understood that naming something you cannot yet explain is an honest acknowledgment of a genuine phenomenon. The grass juice factor was not considered hypothetical. It was empirically observed, reproducible across multiple research groups, and measurable in biological outcomes. Scientists knew something in the juice was exerting protective and regenerative effects. They simply did not yet have the tools to see what it was.

Why Interest Faded, and Why It Shouldn't Have

By the 1950s and into the following decades, the scientific momentum behind the grass juice factor began to slow. This was not because the observations had been disproven or the results called into question. It was because the direction of nutritional science itself was changing.

Isolated vitamins, synthetic supplements, and pharmaceutical compounds became the dominant focus of research. Funding followed patents, and patents required single, identifiable, reproducible molecules. Whole-food bioactive compounds were difficult to study because they could not be easily standardized. They were difficult to patent because they existed in nature. And there was simply not enough financial incentive for large research institutions or pharmaceutical companies to pursue the mysteries of powdered grass juice when more profitable avenues were available.

The grass juice factor became, for several decades, a scientific footnote, a recognized but unresolved observation, sitting quietly in the literature, waiting for better analytical tools and a renewed willingness to ask what whole living food does that no collection of isolated nutrients can replicate.

That waiting, as it turned out, was not in vain. The tools eventually arrived. And what modern analytical chemistry found when it turned its attention back to young barley grass was not a disappointment. It was a vindication, and an explanation far richer than early researchers could have imagined.

A Design Waiting to Be Understood

Looking back at the grass juice factor research with the knowledge available today, what stands out is not the limitation of early science. It is the consistency of what those early scientists observed. Working without HPLC columns, mass spectrometers, or genomic analysis tools, they documented effects that modern research has now begun to explain at the molecular level. The fertility effects, the milk quality findings, and the resilience of animals fed young cereal grasses were not artifacts or errors. They were real observations of a real biological system doing what it was designed to do.

A Creator who embedded that much biological intelligence into a young grass plant (who placed compounds in the juice of barley that support fertility, immune function, metabolic regulation, and cellular repair, and who made those compounds water-soluble so they would concentrate precisely in the juice where they could be most easily consumed) did not do so accidentally. The scientists of the 1930s were observing a design they could not yet name. The scientists of the 21st century are finally learning to read it.

Chapter 3 turns to that reading, to the modern analytical work that identified what the grass juice factor actually contains, corrected a decade-long misidentification, and gave us the biochemical vocabulary to understand why young barley grass juice does what Schnabel and Kohler spent their careers documenting.

IDENTIFYING THE GRASS JUICE FACTOR: THE DETECTIVE WORK BEHIND BARLEY'S FLAVONE PROFILE

For decades, researchers knew that something in young barley grass juice was producing remarkable biological effects. They had named it the grass juice factor. They had measured its influence on fertility, growth, immunity, and resilience across multiple animal models. What they could not do, with the tools available to them, was identify exactly what it was.

That changed gradually, and not without a few wrong turns along the way.

A Promising Lead, and a Mistaken Identity

In 1992, a research team led by Osawa and colleagues published what appeared to be a breakthrough. Working with young green barley leaves, they isolated what they described as a novel antioxidant compound and gave it a name so long it was immediately shortened to an abbreviation: 2"-O-GIV. They classified it as a type of plant compound called an isoflavonoid, and their finding attracted attention. Subsequent papers built on the identification, describing the compound's antioxidant properties and its potential role in protecting against arterial disease.

For nearly a decade, 2"-O-GIV was cited as the key antioxidant in young barley grass. It appeared in nutritional literature, continuing education materials, and product discussions. The identification seemed settled.

It wasn't.

The Correction: Careful Science Rewrites the Record

In 2003, Kenneth Markham and Kevin Mitchell of Industrial Research Ltd. in New Zealand set out to analyze young green barley leaves for a commercial client. Their goal was straightforward: to confirm the presence of 2"-O-GIV. What they found instead stopped them in their tracks.

Using a standard laboratory separation technique, they produced a detailed chemical profile of barley leaf extracts. Two compounds dominated the picture. Neither of them was 2"-O-GIV. To make sure, they obtained a verified sample of authentic 2"-O-GIV and added it directly to the barley extract. When they ran the mixture through the same analysis, the authentic compound separated out in a completely different region, one where the barley extract showed almost nothing.

The original identification was wrong.

Going back to re-examine the data published by Osawa's team a decade earlier, Markham and Mitchell found where the error had occurred. A specific signal in the original chemical fingerprint, one that should have pointed clearly toward the compound's identity, had been misread. It was an honest mistake, the kind that happens when working at the frontier of analytical chemistry, but it had sent the field in the wrong direction for ten years.

What the barley extract actually contained was not a novel compound at all. It was saponarin, a well-characterized plant flavone previously found in mature barley leaves. Markham and Mitchell confirmed this by adding authentic saponarin to the extract and watching the two signals merge perfectly. The second major compound was identified as lutonarin, a close structural relative of saponarin that is commonly found alongside it in barley species.

The detective work was complete. The "novel antioxidant" from barley was neither novel nor the compound that researchers had believed it to be. And importantly, because the original compound had been misclassified as an isoflavonoid, some researchers had speculated it might have estrogen-like activity in the body. Saponarin and lutonarin carry no such concern, a meaningful clarification for anyone consuming barley grass products.

Markham and Mitchell also noted something worth paying attention to: the relative amounts of saponarin and lutonarin in barley leaves can shift depending on how much ultraviolet light the plant receives during growth. This was an early hint that growing conditions matter, a theme that runs throughout this book.

What Saponarin and Lutonarin Actually Are

With the correct identification established, researchers could finally begin to understand what these compounds do.

Saponarin and lutonarin belong to a class of plant compounds called flavone-C-glycosides. The details of that classification matter less than what these compounds do in practice: they are potent antioxidants, capable of neutralizing harmful free radicals that damage cells and accelerate aging and disease. Research has shown their antioxidant activity to be comparable in several test systems to vitamin E, a benchmark most people recognize as meaningful.

Both compounds are water-soluble, which means they concentrate in the juice of the grass rather than remaining locked in the fibrous leaf material. This is not a minor technical detail. It goes directly to why barley grass juice and juice powder behave differently from dried whole-leaf powder. The active compounds are in the juice. More on that in Chapters 9 and 10.

What makes saponarin particularly notable is where it appears in nature. It is found in unusually high concentrations in young barley grass and is largely absent from most other commonly consumed foods. This specificity is part of what makes young barley grass juice biochemically distinctive rather than simply another green vegetable. You are not getting these compounds in meaningful amounts from a salad.

Saponarin Molecular Structure

Of the two, lutonarin is considered the more powerful antioxidant based on its chemical structure. Lutonarin has an arrangement of hydroxyl groups that gives it particularly strong free-radical-scavenging ability. But the two compounds appear to work together, providing complementary coverage rather than competing. This is a theme we will return to: in barley grass juice, compounds rarely work alone.

Lutonarin Molecular Structure

A Third Compound of Interest: Introducing BZ-TMF

More recent research has identified an additional compound in young barley grass that deserves attention: a methylated flavone with the formidable full name 3'-benzyloxy-5,6,7,4'-tetramethoxyflavone, known by the considerably more manageable abbreviation BZ-TMF.

BZ-TMF Molecular Structure

A 2021 study from Cairo University found that BZ-TMF accounts for approximately 49% of the natural plant compounds detected in an analysis of barley grass powder using a sensitive modern technique. That is not a trace amount. It is a dominant constituent within the compounds that particular method captured, suggesting BZ-TMF is not a footnote in the barley grass story but a central character.

Unlike saponarin and lutonarin, whose primary strengths are antioxidant and anti-inflammatory, BZ-TMF appears to influence how the body handles blood sugar and metabolic signaling. This finding provided a biochemical explanation for the previously unexplained observation that barley grass juice improved blood glucose control. BZ-TMF offered a credible mechanism. We will explore this in detail in Chapter 5, where the diabetes and metabolic health research is examined closely.

A Family Resemblance: What Related Flavones Tell Us

BZ-TMF has not yet been studied in isolation in human trials, but it belongs to a well-researched family of methylated flavones, and what that family has shown is worth noting.

Closely related compounds have demonstrated the ability to protect joint cartilage from the kind of cell death that occurs in osteoarthritis. One has shown the ability to reduce lung scarring in animal models of pulmonary fibrosis, a serious and difficult-to-treat condition. Another has been shown to reverse multidrug resistance in cancer cells, essentially making tumors that had become resistant to chemotherapy responsive again. Yet another has demonstrated the ability to reduce a protein that cancer cells use to evade the immune system, a target of significant interest in cancer research.

None of these studies used BZ-TMF directly. But compounds with closely related structures, sharing a common basic framework with similar chemical modifications, tend to exhibit similar biological properties. The presence of BZ-TMF in large amounts in barley grass juice, a compound belonging to a family with this range of documented effects, is not a trivial observation. It is a meaningful piece of the puzzle.

From Mystery to Mechanism, But Not Reductionism

What the work of Markham, Mitchell, and subsequent researchers ultimately revealed was not a single magic molecule. It was a biologically coherent cluster of compounds (saponarin, lutonarin, and BZ-TMF), together capable of explaining many of the effects that early researchers observed but could not account for.

And yet it would be a mistake to conclude that these three flavones are the whole story, or that extracting and concentrating them would replicate what barley grass juice does. The goal here is not to reduce barley grass juice to its most measurable ingredients and discard everything else. The results that people experience, in energy, inflammation, blood sugar, resilience, come from the juice as a whole. The flavones are most meaningful in the context of that complete system, working alongside enzymes, chlorophyll derivatives, minerals, and other cofactors that the plant produces together.

Identifying saponarin, lutonarin, and BZ-TMF gives us a window into the mechanism. It does not give us license to abandon the whole.

In that sense, the detective work of Markham and Mitchell did more than simply correct a mistaken identification. By establishing what was actually present in barley grass, they gave researchers the right target, and in doing so, helped explain why something that scientists first observed in the 1930s was still producing measurable effects in laboratories seventy years later.

The mystery was not solved by finding one thing. It was illuminated by understanding how several things work together, which, it turns out, is exactly how the grass juice factor always worked.

Chapter 4

WHAT MAKES BARLEY GRASS JUICE UNIQUE: ENZYMES, SYNERGY, AND THE LIVING SYSTEM

One of the most revealing details in early barley grass research was not simply what researchers observed, but how they described it. Repeatedly, scientists noted that fresh barley grass juice behaved less like a collection of isolated nutrients and more like a biologically active system. The effects they documented, such as enhanced recovery, improved resilience to stress, and accelerated healing, were difficult to attribute to any single vitamin or mineral.

This was not a vague impression. It was a consistent pattern across multiple research groups working independently. Something about the juice, taken as a whole, produced effects that no single identified component could fully account for. Understanding why requires stepping back from the question of what is in barley grass juice and asking a different question: what kind of thing is it?

Life Produces Living Systems

A young barley plant in its early growth stage is not simply a container of nutrients. It is a metabolically active organism that synthesizes compounds rapidly to support photosynthesis, protect its delicate tissues from oxidative damage, and defend itself against environmental stress. Everything the plant produces during this phase (the enzymes, the flavones, the chlorophyll-related molecules) serves a biological purpose within a coordinated system.

When that juice is extracted carefully and preserved without excessive heat or oxidation, what you capture is not just a list of ingredients. You capture the system itself, or something close to it. This is why early researchers, working with fresh juice, observed effects that later researchers sometimes could not replicate when using processed or whole-leaf preparations. They were working with fundamentally different materials, even when the label said the same thing.

This is also why God's design in the plant kingdom is so remarkable. The compounds in young barley grass were not assembled randomly. They work together in ways that human chemistry has only recently begun to map, and in ways that isolated supplements have never been able to replicate. Life comes from life, and a living plant system, carefully preserved, carries something that a bottle of extracted compounds simply does not.

The Role of Enzymes

Among the most important, and most fragile, components of young barley grass juice are its enzymes.

Enzymes are biological catalysts. They make chemical reactions happen faster and more efficiently than they otherwise would. Every living cell depends on them. In a young barley plant, enzymes are working at high levels to manage the intense metabolic activity of early growth: synthesizing protective compounds, managing oxidative stress generated by rapid photosynthesis, and repairing cellular damage as it occurs.

Many of these enzymes are transient by nature. They exist to serve a specific purpose during a specific developmental window and decline as the plant matures. This means that fresh, young barley grass contains enzymatic activity that older grass simply does not.

When juice is extracted from young barley grass and dried carefully, with minimal heat and protection from oxygen, much of this enzymatic activity can be preserved. When it is processed aggressively, with high heat or prolonged air exposure, the enzymes are among the first things destroyed.

This matters for two reasons.

First, the enzymes themselves contribute to the biological activity of the juice. Antioxidant enzyme systems present in young barley grass help neutralize reactive oxygen species, the unstable molecules that damage cells, accelerate aging, and contribute to chronic disease. While these enzymes are not absorbed into the bloodstream the way vitamins are, research suggests they exert meaningful effects locally in the digestive tract and influence signaling pathways beyond it.

Second, and perhaps more practically, enzymatic activity functions as a quality signal. If a barley grass juice powder retains measurable enzyme activity, it tells you something important about how it was processed. Enzymes are fragile. Their survival is evidence that the processing was gentle enough to preserve other delicate compounds, such as flavones, chlorophyll derivatives, and the full complement of bioactive constituents that make the juice what it is.

If the enzymes are gone, you have reason to wonder what else didn't survive.

Synergy: Why the Whole Is Greater Than the Sum

The concept of synergy is often invoked loosely in nutrition discussions, but in the case of barley grass juice it has genuine scientific grounding.

Flavones like saponarin, lutonarin, and BZ-TMF do not operate in isolation. Their activity is shaped by the biochemical environment in which they exist: the presence of cofactors, the activity of enzyme systems, and the availability of chlorophyll-related molecules that influence how compounds are absorbed and utilized. Change that environment significantly, and the activity changes with it.

This helps explain a persistent frustration in nutritional research: why attempts to isolate the "active ingredient" from whole foods so often produce disappointing results. A compound extracted from its natural context and tested alone frequently underperforms compared to the whole food from which it came. The context is not incidental. It is part of the mechanism.

For barley grass juice, this means that the goal is not to identify the single most important flavone and concentrate it into a capsule. The goal is to preserve the juice, the whole juice, in a form that retains as much of the original living system as possible. Saponarin, lutonarin, and BZ-TMF are important because they help us understand why barley grass juice does what it does. They are not important because they should be extracted and sold separately.

The grass juice factor, as early researchers understood it, was never reducible to one thing. It was the product of a system. Modern analytical chemistry has given us a clearer view of what that system contains. It has not given us reason to abandon the system itself.

The Harvest Window: Why Timing Affects What You Get

Young barley grass undergoes rapid biochemical changes during early growth. In the juvenile stage, the plant is focused on leaf development and cellular protection, synthesizing large quantities of antioxidant compounds, flavones, and enzymes to meet the demands of rapid growth.

As the plant matures and approaches what agronomists call the jointing stage, the point at which stem elongation begins, the plant's priorities shift. Resources are redirected from leaf protection toward structural growth and eventual seed formation. Flavone concentrations decline. Enzymatic activity decreases. The grass may still look green and healthy, but its biochemical profile has changed significantly.

This matters primarily for understanding inconsistencies in the research record. Studies that used barley grass harvested before this transition tend to show stronger biological effects than those that may have used more mature material. It is one reason why results across different research groups are not always directly comparable.

The material being studied was not always equivalent, even when it carried the same name.

For consumers, the practical implication is simpler: harvest timing is one of several variables that responsible producers control, and it is worth understanding that "barley grass" on a label does not guarantee a consistent biochemical profile. What is inside the package depends heavily on decisions made in the field and in the processing facility, decisions that are not visible from the outside of the container.

Field-Grown vs. Tray-Grown: A Distinction That Matters Before Processing Begins

Harvest timing is not the only growing variable that determines what ends up in a barley grass product. The method and environment in which the grass is grown matter just as much, and this distinction is worth understanding because it affects the raw material before any processing decision is made.

Ronald Seibold, in his foundational work *Cereal Grass: Nature's Greatest Gift*, drew a careful distinction between cereal grass grown in outdoor fields through a full growing cycle and the quickly sprouted "wheatgrass" grown indoors on trays and cut within five to seven days. The difference is not merely one of convenience or scale. It is biochemical.

Field-grown cereal grasses such as barley, wheat, rye, or oats planted in the fall and grown for roughly 200 days through the cold months pass through multiple developmental stages that tray-grown sprouts never reach. The cold growing season, the deep root development, the soil mineral uptake, and the slow accumulation of photosynthetic activity are all necessary for the plant to convert simple sugars into the complex organic molecules that define nutritionally potent cereal grass. Chlorophyll, protein, enzymes, and the flavone compounds discussed throughout this book reach their peak concentrations in the period just before the jointing stage, a milestone that tray-grown grass, cut in less than a week, never approaches.

Tray-grown wheatgrass is not without value. It contains chlorophyll and some nutritional benefits, and it has been used therapeutically by many practitioners. But as Seibold observed, it is more accurately described as a long sprout than a fully developed grass. It lacks the enzyme systems and the complex nutrient profile that develop only when the plant passes through the environmental conditions and growth stages that outdoor field cultivation provides. The simple sugars produced by its brief photosynthesis are never converted into the organic molecules that make field-grown cereal grass what it is.

This matters practically because both products are often sold under similar names and positioned similarly in the marketplace. A juice made from tray-grown wheatgrass and a powder made from field-grown barley grass harvested just before the jointing stage are not equivalent products, even if both are green, both are raw, and both are marketed as cereal grass juice. The ceiling of what tray-grown grass can deliver is lower, not because of how it was processed, but because of what it never had the opportunity to become.

The best barley grass juice powders begin with field-grown grass, cultivated in mineral-rich soil, grown through the cool seasons that drive biochemical complexity, and harvested at precisely the right developmental moment. Everything that follows (the juicing, the low-temperature drying, the cold storage) is an effort to preserve what that carefully grown plant produced. No amount of careful processing can compensate for starting with a raw material that never reached its full biochemical potential.

Why Some Products Work and Others Disappoint

When people try barley grass products and find them unhelpful, the explanation is rarely that barley grass itself is ineffective. It is more often the case that the product they used no longer resembles the biologically active material that researchers studied.

Processing is the critical variable. A powder can look vibrant green and still be biochemically compromised. Color tells you very little about what survived the journey from field to jar. What you want to know is whether the water-soluble flavones were concentrated through juice extraction, whether the processing was gentle enough to preserve enzymatic activity, and whether the product came from grass harvested at the right developmental stage.

These are not marketing questions. They are scientific ones, and they have answers if producers are willing to be transparent about how their products are made and tested.

We will examine exactly how to evaluate these questions in Chapters 9 and 10, where the differences between juice powder and whole-leaf powder are laid out clearly, and where independent testing data provide a concrete basis for comparison.

For now, the essential point is this: barley grass juice is not simply a green powder. It is a living system, captured at a specific moment in a plant's development and preserved through careful handling. When that system is intact, the results that early researchers observed, and that modern laboratory studies continue to document, become possible. When it is compromised, those results become unlikely, regardless of what the label claims.

Chapter 5

METABOLIC HEALTH AND DIABETES: WHAT THE RESEARCH ACTUALLY SHOWS

Diabetes is a relentless disease. Elevated blood sugar, damaged kidneys, failing eyesight, painful neuropathy in the feet, increased risk of heart disease, slow-healing wounds, and a shortened life are not rare complications. They are the expected trajectory for millions of people who cannot reliably control their blood glucose. For those searching for natural tools to support their health alongside conventional care, the research on barley grass juice and metabolic function offers something genuinely worth examining.

The connection between barley grass juice and metabolic health did not emerge from abstract theory. It arose from controlled experimental work examining how barley grass juice affects glucose handling, insulin sensitivity, oxidative stress, and organ protection, the key drivers and consequences of diabetes progression.

Blood Sugar Control: What Animal Studies Show

One of the clearest demonstrations comes from a study published in *Heliyon* in 2019 by Mohamed and colleagues, who investigated the effects of barley grass juice in rats with experimentally induced diabetes. Diabetic rats given barley grass juice daily showed significant reductions in fasting blood glucose compared with untreated diabetic controls. They also demonstrated improved lipid profiles and boosted antioxidant enzyme activity, suggesting that barley grass juice was not merely lowering blood sugar but reducing the oxidative stress that drives diabetes complications at the cellular level.

What made this finding particularly relevant was the absence of hypoglycemia. Blood glucose improved without dropping below normal ranges. This matters because it reinforces the idea that barley grass juice supports metabolic regulation rather than forcing glucose down pharmacologically, a meaningful distinction for anyone managing diabetes alongside other treatments.

A Deeper Look: The Eight-Group Study

A more comprehensive picture emerged from a 2021 study published in *Experimental Biology and Medicine* by Mohamed, Abdel-Rahim, Aly, Naguib, and Khattab, along with a companion 2022 paper in *Food Science & Nutrition* examining reproductive outcomes in the same animals. These studies used barley microgreens, young barley grass harvested at peak nutritional density, and designed an unusually thorough experimental model.

The researchers divided rats into eight groups, creating conditions that ranged from healthy controls to worst-case scenarios combining induced diabetes with aflatoxin B1 exposure. Aflatoxin is a toxic mold compound that compounds metabolic damage, making it a useful stress test for any protective intervention. The groups were:
- G1: Healthy controls
- G2: Barley microgreens only
- G3: Aflatoxin only
- G4: Aflatoxin plus barley microgreens
- G5: Induced diabetes (STZ) only
- G6: Induced diabetes plus barley microgreens
- G7: Induced diabetes plus aflatoxin
- G8: Induced diabetes plus aflatoxin plus barley microgreens

The results across blood sugar, pancreatic function, organ health, and antioxidant status were striking enough to warrant presenting the data directly.

Blood Glucose Results

The data tells a clear story. Healthy controls (G1) maintained blood glucose around 100 mg/dL. Diabetic rats without intervention (G5) rose to 150 mg/dL. Adding barley microgreens to the diabetic group (G6) reduced it to 124 mg/dL, a meaningful reduction. The most severe group (diabetes combined with aflatoxin (G7)) reached 176 mg/dL, and even here, barley microgreens (G8) pulled blood glucose back to 150 mg/dL, matching the level of the untreated diabetic group. In other words, barley microgreens entirely offset the additional metabolic damage caused by aflatoxin exposure.

Notably, barley microgreens given to healthy rats (G2) resulted in a blood glucose level of 99 mg/dL, essentially identical to that of healthy controls, confirming that the effect is regulatory rather than indiscriminate glucose suppression.

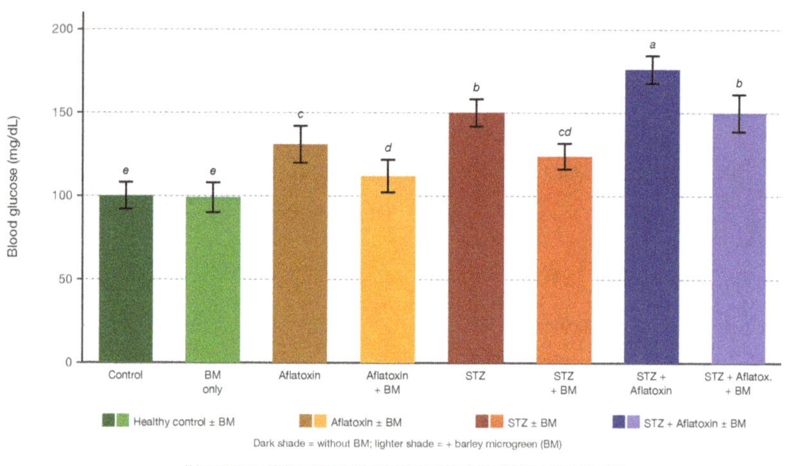

Figure 5.1 Blood Glucose Results from 8 Group Rat Study. Data from Mohamed et al 2022.

Pancreatic Beta Cell Preservation

Perhaps the most visually compelling finding concerned the insulin-producing beta cells of the pancreas, which diabetes progressively destroys.

In healthy controls (G1), approximately 17.5% of pancreatic islet tissue stained positive for insulin, reflecting a robust population of functioning beta cells. In untreated diabetic rats (G5), that figure collapsed to roughly 4%, a devastating loss of insulin-producing capacity. When barley microgreens were added to the diabetic group (G6), the beta cell area recovered to approximately 12%, nearly three times that of untreated diabetic animals.

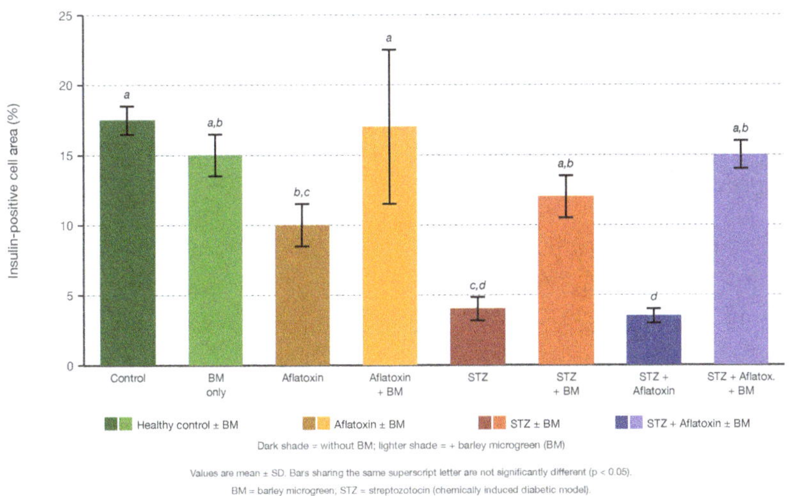

Figure 5.2 Insulin-Positive Beta-Cells Protected by Barley Microgreens. Data from Mohamed et al 2022

The worst outcome was observed in rats exposed to both diabetes and aflatoxin (G7), with the beta-cell area falling to approximately 3.5%. Adding barley microgreens to this group (G8) restored beta cell area to roughly 15%, exceeding the recovery seen in the diabetic-only treated group and approaching healthy control levels.

These are not trivial differences. Preserving beta cells is one of the central challenges in diabetes management. The finding that barley microgreens supported meaningful recovery of insulin-producing tissue, even under the compound stress of diabetes and a potent environmental toxin, points to a protective mechanism operating at a fundamental level.

The companion 2022 study documented additional benefits in the same animals, including improved insulin sensitivity, reduced markers of insulin resistance, and protection of the liver, kidneys, and reproductive tissues from diabetes- and aflatoxin-induced damage. Diabetic male rats showed improved sperm health and reduced testicular damage, a lesser-known but significant complication of poorly controlled diabetes, with barley microgreen supplementation partially reversing these effects.

The High-Fat Diet Study: Weight, Cholesterol, and Vascular Protection

A separate animal study took a different angle, examining whether barley grass juice could protect against the broader metabolic damage caused by a high-fat diet. Researchers divided rats into five groups: healthy controls, a high-fat diet group, a high-fat diet group treated with atorvastatin (a commonly prescribed statin drug), and two high-fat diet groups receiving different doses of barley grass juice (200 mg/kg and 400 mg/kg per day) over 60 days.

The results were striking across every measured outcome:

- Abnormal weight gain was substantially reduced in rats receiving barley grass juice powder at the higher dose, despite consuming the same high-fat diet as the untreated obese group.
- Cholesterol levels were normalized, performing as well as or better than the statin-treated group.

- Liver enzymes, markers of fatty liver injury, remained within normal ranges.
- Carotid artery tissue examined under the microscope appeared near-normal despite high-fat diet exposure.
- Antioxidant enzyme systems in the liver, including catalase, superoxide dismutase, and reduced glutathione, were restored to healthy levels.
- Lipid peroxidation, the oxidative damage that accelerates arterial disease, remained low and comparable to that of healthy controls.

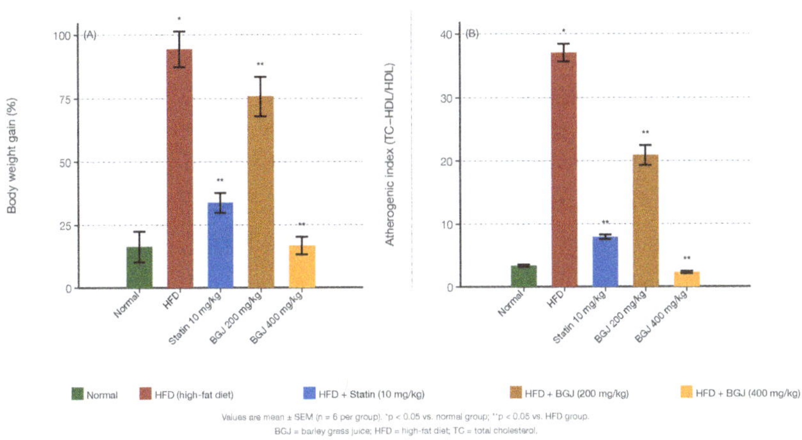

Figure 5.3 Barley Grass Juice Protects Against High-Fat Diet in Animal Study. Data from Thatiparthi et al (2019).

Two molecular markers deserve particular attention. PPAR-gamma, a protein elevated in obesity and implicated in fat accumulation, was normalized despite the high-fat diet. Caspase-3, a marker of cell death that rises in metabolically damaged tissue, was also normalized. These findings suggest that barley grass juice powder was interacting with metabolism at a signaling level. It was not merely absorbing fat or blocking its digestion, but influencing the molecular machinery that governs how cells respond to metabolic stress.

That a whole-food product matched or exceeded a pharmaceutical statin on several of these measurements is notable, though it should be interpreted carefully. Rats are not people, doses do not translate directly, and no one should abandon prescribed medications based on animal research. But the consistency of these findings across multiple metabolic markers is difficult to dismiss.

The Mechanism: Where BZ-TMF Fits In

Earlier research on the effects of barley grass juice in diabetic models produced encouraging results but offered a limited explanation of how the juice worked. The identification of BZ-TMF, introduced in Chapter 3, provided a credible answer.

Research has shown that BZ-TMF influences the pathways that control how much glucose the liver produces and releases into the bloodstream. In type 2 diabetes, the liver tends to overproduce glucose, contributing significantly to elevated fasting blood sugar levels. BZ-TMF appears to modulate the enzymes involved in this process, reducing excess glucose output and improving the liver's responsiveness to insulin signaling.

This is not the same as a drug forcing glucose down. It is a compound that works with existing metabolic pathways to restore a balance disrupted by diabetes. That distinction matters both mechanistically and practically.

Given that BZ-TMF accounts for a significant proportion of the phytochemicals detected in barley grass powder by one analysis, and given that it concentrates in the juice fraction rather than the fibrous leaf, it represents a compelling explanation for why barley grass juice powder produces the metabolic effects observed in these studies, and why whole-leaf preparations are less likely to deliver equivalent results.

What This Means, and What It Doesn't

These studies were conducted in rats, not people. The diabetic model used, streptozotocin injection, creates a rapid-onset diabetes that differs in important ways from the chronic, lifestyle-driven type 2 diabetes that affects most people. Dose equivalencies between rat studies and human intake cannot be calculated directly. Human clinical trials are needed before any of these findings can be translated into specific recommendations.

What the research does provide is a biologically credible rationale. The mechanisms identified (beta-cell protection, hepatic glucose regulation, antioxidant system support, and lipid normalization) are relevant to human diabetes. The compounds responsible, particularly BZ-TMF, saponarin, and lutonarin, are present in well-made barley grass juice powder. The consistency of results across multiple independent studies examining different aspects of metabolic function suggests that something real is happening rather than a statistical artifact.

For anyone managing diabetes or metabolic syndrome, barley grass juice powder is not a replacement for medical care, dietary discipline, or prescribed treatment. It is a whole-food addition with a growing body of evidence suggesting it supports the body's own metabolic regulatory systems in ways that isolated vitamins and minerals do not.

God designed plants to serve our health in ways we are still discovering. The evidence on barley grass juice and metabolic function is one of the clearer examples of that design revealing itself through careful scientific inquiry.

Chapter 6

MENTAL HEALTH, FATIGUE, AND STRESS: EVIDENCE BEYOND MOOD CHEMISTRY

Depression is one of the most common and most difficult conditions people face. It affects millions worldwide, cuts across age and background, and resists simple solutions. For many people, the search for relief is genuinely desperate, and pharmaceutical antidepressants, whatever their limitations, offer something that desperate people need: a result they can feel, quickly enough to keep going.

This should not be overlooked. When someone is in crisis, stabilization matters. A pharmaceutical medication can provide the footing a person needs while deeper, slower work begins. Natural foods and plant-based approaches work differently, more gradually, more fundamentally, and they need time to take effect. For someone in acute distress, that timeline is not always workable on its own.

What the research on barley grass juice suggests is not that it replaces pharmaceutical treatment. It suggests that it may support the underlying biological environment in which the nervous system operates by reducing oxidative stress in brain tissue, promoting the production of neuroprotective factors, and improving cellular resilience to stress. These are not the same mechanisms that antidepressants target, which is precisely why they may be complementary rather than competing approaches.

Why Oxidative Stress Matters for Mental Health

The relationship between nutrition and mental health is often reduced to neurotransmitter science, such as serotonin levels, dopamine pathways, and chemical imbalances. But this picture, while familiar, is increasingly recognized as incomplete. A growing body of research points to oxidative stress and neuroinflammation as significant contributors to depression, anxiety, and fatigue.

The brain is exceptionally vulnerable to oxidative damage. It accounts for roughly 20% of the body's oxygen consumption despite representing only about 2% of body weight. That intense metabolic activity generates substantial quantities of free radicals, and the brain's high lipid content makes it particularly susceptible to oxidative injury. When antioxidant defenses are overwhelmed by chronic stress, poor nutrition, environmental toxins, or illness, the result is measurable damage to neurons and the signaling systems they depend on.

This is where barley grass juice enters the picture. The flavones concentrated in young barley grass juice (saponarin, lutonarin, and BZ-TMF) are potent antioxidants with demonstrated ability to protect cells from oxidative damage. Whether they can do the same in brain tissue is what a series of animal studies set out to examine.

Study 1: Barley and Wheat Grass Extracts Help Mice Handle Stress-Induced Depression

The first line of evidence comes from a 2022 study published in the *Journal of Ayurveda and Integrative Medicine* by researchers in Kathmandu, Nepal. Barley grass products had become popular in Nepal, and this study was motivated in part by the desire to understand why. The researchers investigated aqueous extracts from both barley and wheat grass in Swiss albino mice subjected to stress-induced depression.

Mice were divided into groups and exposed to stress conditions. They received either the grass extracts at 400 mg/kg, a standard antidepressant drug called imipramine, or a control. Behavioral tests included three established methods for measuring despair, immobility, and anxiety in animal models: the forced swim test, the tail suspension test, and the elevated plus maze.

The extracts contained significant quantities of alkaloids, flavonoids, phenols, and tannins, with strong antioxidant activity measured across multiple test systems. In behavioral testing, treated mice showed significantly reduced immobility time in both the forced swim and tail suspension tests, and spent more time in the open arms of the elevated plus maze, indicating reduced anxiety and depression-like behavior compared to stressed control animals.

The researchers concluded that the antioxidant polyphenols and flavonoids naturally present in these grasses were likely responsible for the antidepressant-like activity. The effect was meaningful, reproducible, and comparable in direction, if not identical in magnitude, to the pharmaceutical control.

Study 2: Barley Leaf Extract and the Brain's Stress Response

A Japanese research group at Chiba University published findings in 2012 in *Pharmacognosy Research* that examined what barley leaf extract was doing in the brain during stress. Using the forced swimming test (in which immobility duration serves as a proxy for behavioral despair), they gave mice either barley leaf extract at 400 or 1000 mg/kg, imipramine, or a control, one hour before swimming sessions over three days.

Both doses of barley leaf extract significantly reduced immobility time, producing an antidepressant-like effect comparable in direction to imipramine. But the more interesting finding came from the biochemical analysis. The researchers measured gene expression in the hippocampus and cortex, specifically focusing on nerve growth factor (NGF), brain-derived neurotrophic factor (BDNF), and glucocorticoid receptor (GR) levels.

Stress increased NGF expression in the hippocampus by 31%. Barley leaf extract moderated this response in a dose-dependent manner, suggesting it influenced the brain's own stress signaling rather than simply sedating the animals. Importantly, motor activity remained normal throughout, and the mice were not tranquilized. The effect appeared to be genuine stress resilience rather than pharmacological suppression.

Serum corticosterone, the primary stress hormone, was unchanged by the extract, suggesting that barley leaf was not interfering with the body's stress hormone axis directly. The researchers proposed instead that its effects involved modulating neurotrophic signaling in the brain, potentially offering neuroprotection against the cumulative damage of chronic stress.

Study 3: Preserving Brain Health Under Repeated Stress

The same Chiba University research group published a follow-up study in 2015 in *Pharmacognosy Magazine*, this time examining the ability of young green barley leaves to protect against repeated restraint stress in female mice. Rather than a single behavioral test, this study tracked voluntary wheel-running activity over five days of stress exposure, a measure of motivation and adaptive capacity that reliably declines under chronic stress.

Mice underwent three hours of restraint stress daily for five days. Those given barley leaf extract at 400 or 1000 mg/kg beforehand showed significantly better preservation of wheel-running activity compared to stressed controls. They were more willing to move, explore, and engage, the behavioral signature of an animal that has maintained some resilience against stress rather than succumbing to it.

The biochemical findings supported this picture. Stress reduced hippocampal BDNF, the brain's key neuroprotective growth factor, often found at lower levels in people with depression, and barley leaf extract, particularly at the 400 mg/kg dose, significantly preserved BDNF expression, including a specific variant called exon IV, which is particularly important for long-term neuronal health.

Again, corticosterone levels were unaffected, and non-stressed mice given the extract showed no hyperactivity or abnormal behavior. The effect was protective rather than stimulating, exactly the kind of response you would hope to see from a nutritional intervention rather than a drug.

Fatigue and Physical Resilience

Beyond mood and stress, cereal grass extracts have been examined directly in the context of chronic fatigue, one of the most debilitating and poorly understood conditions affecting people today, and one that sits at the intersection of mental, neurological, and metabolic health.

A 2014 study by Borah, Sarma, and Das at Assam Medical College in India, published in *Pharmacognosy Research*, investigated the effects of wheatgrass extract in a validated animal model of chronic fatigue syndrome. Mice were subjected to forced swimming for six minutes daily over seven days, a protocol reliably shown to produce a CFS-like state characterized by progressive exhaustion, anxiety, and reduced motivation to move. Five groups were studied: a naive control, a stressed control, two groups receiving wheatgrass extract at 100 and 200 mg/kg, and a group receiving imipramine as a pharmaceutical reference.

The stressed control animals showed exactly what the model predicts: increasing immobility over the seven days, reduced locomotor activity in open-field testing, elevated anxiety in both the elevated plus maze and mirror chamber tests, and biochemical evidence of oxidative stress in brain tissue, namely decreased catalase activity and increased malondialdehyde, a marker of lipid peroxidation.

Wheatgrass extract reversed all of these changes in a dose-dependent manner. Treated animals showed progressively less immobility as the week progressed, the opposite of the trajectory observed in stressed controls (See Figure 6.1). Locomotor activity recovered significantly. Anxiety measures improved. And critically, catalase activity in the brain increased while malondialdehyde levels fell, indicating that the extract directly reduced the oxidative burden on brain tissue imposed by the chronic stress protocol.

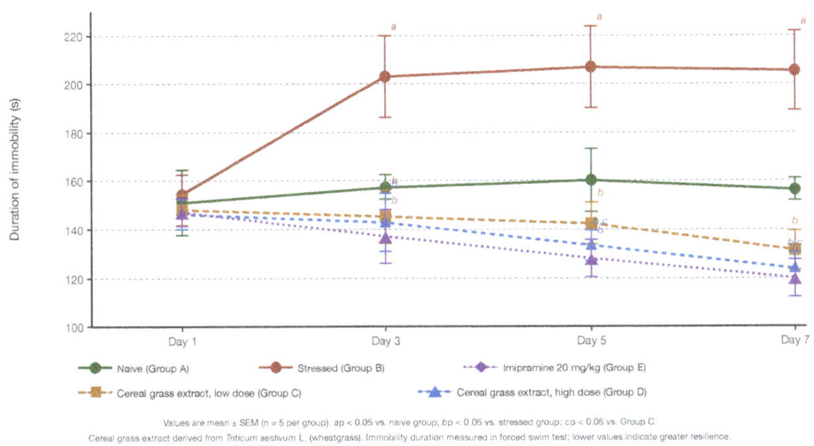

Figure 6.1 Cereal Grass Extract Helps with Fatigue and Immobility.
Data from Borah, Sarma, and Das, 2014.

The effects were comparable in direction to imipramine, the pharmaceutical control, without producing sedation or abnormal behavior. The researchers attributed the activity to the flavonoid content of wheatgrass, specifically apigenin, quercetin, and luteolin, which share structural and functional similarities with saponarin and lutonarin, which are found at high concentrations in young barley grass.

This study matters for the barley grass story because it confirms that the fatigue-protective effects of cereal grass juice are not isolated to a single species or a single research group. The same family of compounds, in a closely related plant, protects brain tissue from oxidative stress-driven fatigue through measurable, reproducible biochemical mechanisms.

For people dealing with the exhaustion that so often accompanies chronic illness, depression, or stress overload, these findings are directly relevant. Fatigue is rarely purely psychological. It has a cellular foundation, and that foundation is where cereal grass flavones appear to exert their deepest influence.

What These Studies Tell Us, and What They Don't

These are animal studies, and that limitation matters. Depression in people is far more complex than stress-induced behavioral changes in mice. The doses used in animal research do not translate directly to human intake. The models of stress used (forced swimming, tail suspension, and physical restraint) are imperfect proxies for the lived experience of human depression, anxiety, and chronic fatigue.

What these studies do provide is a biologically plausible mechanism. The brain is an organ under constant oxidative pressure. The neuroprotective growth factors that sustain it (NGF, BDNF) are sensitive to that pressure and decline under chronic stress. The flavones in barley grass juice have demonstrated antioxidant activity in brain tissue and the ability to modulate the very signaling pathways involved in stress resilience and neuroprotection.

That is not a cure for depression. It is a foundation, one that supports the biological environment in which healing, whether through natural means or pharmaceutical assistance, becomes more possible.

For anyone searching for natural tools to complement their mental health journey, barley grass juice powder is not a replacement for professional care or, when needed, medication. It is a whole-food support that works gradually and deeply, giving the nervous system what it needs to do what God designed it to do: adapt, recover, and heal.

Chapter 7

CANCER RESEARCH AND CELLULAR PROTECTION: WHAT LABORATORY STUDIES TELL US

Cancer is one of the most feared words in any language. For people under the age of 65 in the United States, it is the leading cause of death. Most of us have watched someone we love face it, and we know that the experience is rarely simple, rarely predictable, and rarely resolved by any single treatment.

That complexity matters for how we read the research on barley grass juice and cancer. The studies that exist are real, the findings are meaningful, and they deserve careful attention. But they need to be understood for what they are (early-stage laboratory and animal evidence pointing toward biological mechanisms) not as proof that barley grass juice treats or cures cancer. That distinction is not a legal disclaimer. It is an honest reflection of where the science stands.

What the research does suggest is that barley grass juice contains compounds that support the body's own cellular defense systems: protecting DNA from damage, slowing the growth of cancer cells under controlled conditions, and strengthening the immune responses that identify and eliminate abnormal cells. In the context of a genuinely holistic approach to cancer, this is beneficial. But on its own, it is not enough.

Understanding Cancer Holistically

Before examining the research, it is worth stepping back to acknowledge what cancer actually is and what is required to address it.

Cancer does not arise in a vacuum. It develops in a biological environment compromised by chronic inflammation, oxidative stress, immune dysfunction, metabolic disruption, and often years of accumulated cellular damage. It is also, for many people, preceded or accompanied by an emotional and spiritual crisis. Practitioners who work closely with cancer patients frequently observe a significant emotional event, such as a loss, a prolonged period of unresolved stress, or a deep wound in the period before diagnosis. Whether this is causal or correlational remains an open question scientifically, but it points to the reality that cancer touches a person at every level of their being, not just the cellular one.

This means that addressing cancer well requires an all-hands-on-deck approach. Diet matters. A whole-foods, plant-rich diet reduces the inflammatory and metabolic conditions that allow cancer to thrive. Sleep matters. The body's repair systems are most active during deep sleep, and chronic sleep deprivation impairs immune surveillance. Physical activity matters. It improves immune function, reduces inflammatory signaling, and supports the metabolic health that cancer disrupts. Stress management matters. Chronic stress elevates cortisol, suppresses immune activity, and creates the biological environment in which cancer finds its footing. And emotional and spiritual health matter. Unresolved grief, fear, anger, and isolation are not separate from the body. They live in it.

Barley grass juice powder is a small but meaningful part of this larger picture. The research that follows describes what it may contribute, not what it can do alone.

Laboratory Studies: Barley Grass Extracts and Cancer Cells

The most extensive body of laboratory research on barley grass and cancer comes from a research group at the Institute of Rural Health in Lublin, Poland, which conducted a series of cell culture studies examining barley grass extracts against multiple cancer cell lines.

In a 2019 study, researchers tested water-based extracts from both dried whole-leaf barley grass powder and dehydrated juice powder on LS180 and HT-29 colon cancer cell lines as well as normal human colon cells. The extracts did not harm normal cell growth or structure but significantly reduced the proliferation of colon cancer cells. Higher doses produced stronger effects, and microscopic examination showed signs of necrosis (cell death) in the cancer cells. The authors noted that the dehydrated juice powder was a more effective anti-proliferative agent than the dried whole leaf powder, consistent with the argument throughout this book that the active compounds concentrate in the juice fraction.

A 2017 study from the same group tested similar extracts against HT-29 colon cancer cells and A549 lung cancer cells, again showing low toxicity to normal cells alongside meaningful reductions in cancer cell growth. Flavonoids were identified as likely contributors to the observed activity.

A 2020 study took the investigation a step further by combining barley grass with chlorella (a green algae with its own established research record) against HT-29 colon cancer cells. The barley extract alone slowed cancer cell growth and caused necrosis-like changes while sparing normal cells. The combination of barley grass and chlorella outperformed either ingredient alone, though not in a fully additive way. This kind of interaction, where two natural compounds work better together than separately, is common in phytochemical research and reflects the same synergy principle discussed in Chapter 4. Nutrients are team players. They rarely act as silver bullets.

In 2023, the same synergy was observed in a study focused on breast cancer cells, specifically the T47D cell line. Barley grass water extract increased cancer cell membrane permeability and reduced growth, with signs of necrosis. When paired with chlorella, the combination was more effective than either alone and did not affect normal skin cells.

Taken together, this series of four studies from a single research group, each examining different cancer cell types and experimental conditions, consistently points to the same conclusion: barley grass extracts can slow cancer cell growth and promote cell death under controlled laboratory conditions, while leaving normal cells relatively unaffected. That selectivity is important. It suggests that the compounds interact with something specific to cancer cell biology rather than simply being toxic to all cells.

Animal Studies: Immune Activation and Tumor Reduction

Laboratory cell studies are useful for understanding mechanisms, but animal studies move the evidence closer to biological reality. Two animal studies add important dimensions to the cancer picture.

A 2023 study examined mice with hepatocellular carcinoma (liver cancer) in which tumors were triggered using a gene-delivery method. Some mice received barley grass juice as a supplement. The results showed that barley grass juice reduced tumor growth, and the mechanism appeared to involve immune activation rather than direct tumor toxicity. Tests revealed higher levels of immune markers, including CD45 and F4/80, indicating increased infiltration of immune cells, particularly macrophages, into tumor tissue. Barley grass juice appeared to be helping the immune system recognize and respond to early-stage tumors, which is precisely the kind of immune surveillance that cancer disrupts.

A 2016 study in mice with experimentally induced breast cancer found that barley grass powder slowed carcinogenesis in a dose-dependent manner. Deeper analysis of the cell culture component of the same study identified the flavones lutonarin and saponarin as responsible for a significant portion of the observed benefit, the first study to directly implicate these specific compounds in cancer-related activity.

Natural Killer Cells: Strengthening the Body's First Responders

A 2022 study from the Lublin research group added another dimension, one focused not on cancer cells directly but on the immune cells that hunt them.

Natural killer cells, commonly called NK cells, are front-line immune defenders. Unlike other immune cells that require prior exposure to an antigen before responding, NK cells can recognize and destroy abnormal cells, including cancer cells, without prior activation. They are among the body's most important first responders against early tumor development.

In this study, barley grass extract was found to boost NK cell activity against colon cancer cells. The direct anti-proliferative effect of the extract on cancer cells was modest in this experimental setup, as seen in the light (green) bars in Figure 7.1. The enhancement of NK cell function was the more significant finding, shown in the dark (green) hashed bars in Figure 7.1. This points to a mechanism that operates through immune empowerment rather than direct cytotoxicity, which is biologically meaningful because a well-functioning immune system is the body's most sophisticated and adaptive defense against cancer.

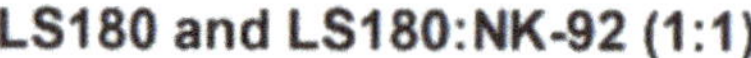

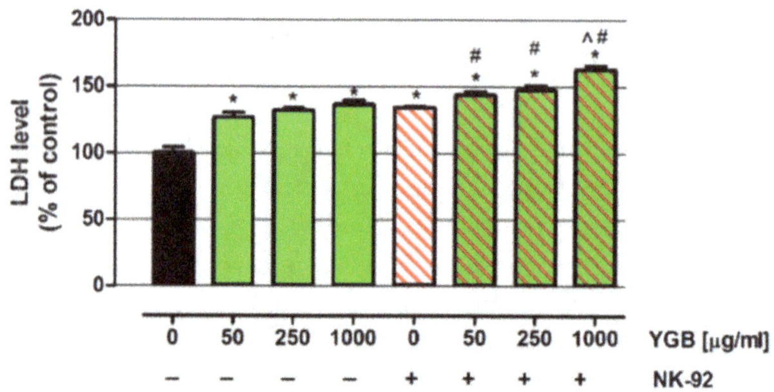

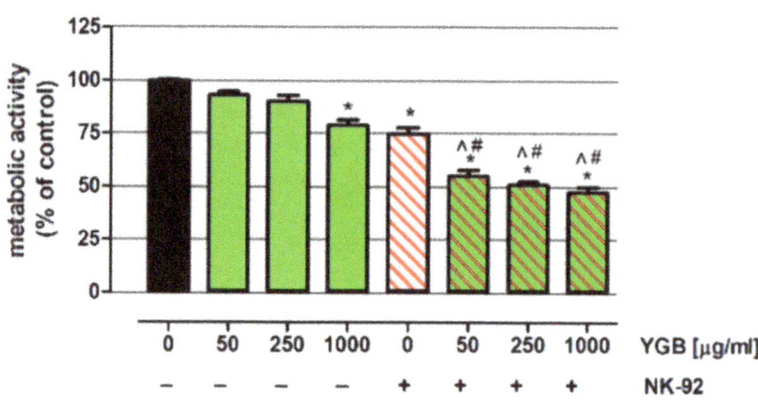

Figure 7.1 Young Green Barley Extract (YGB) impact on NK-92 cell cytotoxicity. LDH is a measure of cell death. Reduced metabolic activity indicates cell death. From Lemieszek et all 2022.

DNA Protection: The Preventive Argument

Beyond its effects on existing cancer cells, barley grass juice has been studied for its ability to protect healthy cells from the DNA damage that initiates cancer.

In 2009, a study commissioned by Hallelujah Diet was conducted at the Cancer Chemoprotection Core Laboratory of the Linus Pauling Institute at Oregon State University, which is one of the world's leading micronutrient research centers. Researcher David Yu, Ph.D., used the comet assay, a sensitive and well-validated technique for measuring DNA strand breaks in individual cells, to determine whether BarleyMax, a premium barley grass juice powder produced by low-temperature drying, could protect human colon cells from oxidative DNA damage.

The results were clear and reproducible across two independent experiments. When colon cancer cells were exposed to an oxidative stressor in the presence of increasing concentrations of BarleyMax, DNA damage declined in a dose-dependent manner. At higher concentrations, cells were almost completely protected. The damage was reduced to approximately 10% of the level seen without Barley-Max. Both experiments showed statistically significant protection at every dose level tested.

As with all in vitro research, these results cannot be directly applied to DNA protection in living people. But similar in vitro findings with kiwifruit juice, broccoli sprouts, spinach, and carrot juice have shown meaningful correlation with DNA protection measured in human volunteers, suggesting the biological pattern is real and worth taking seriously.

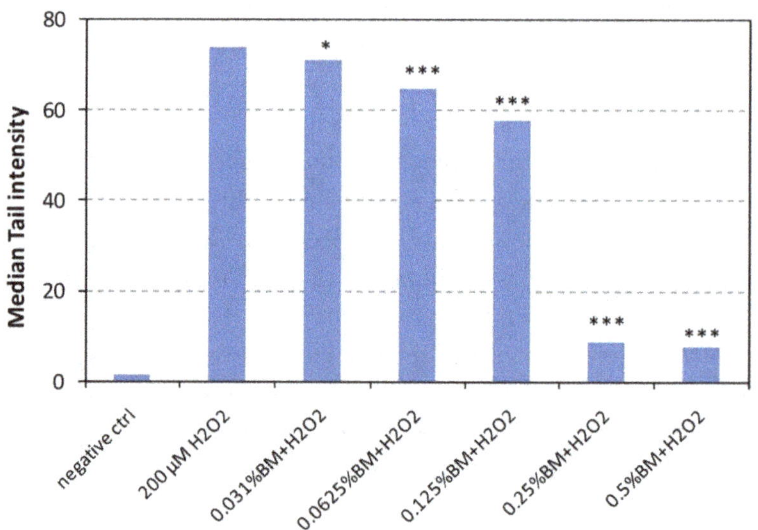

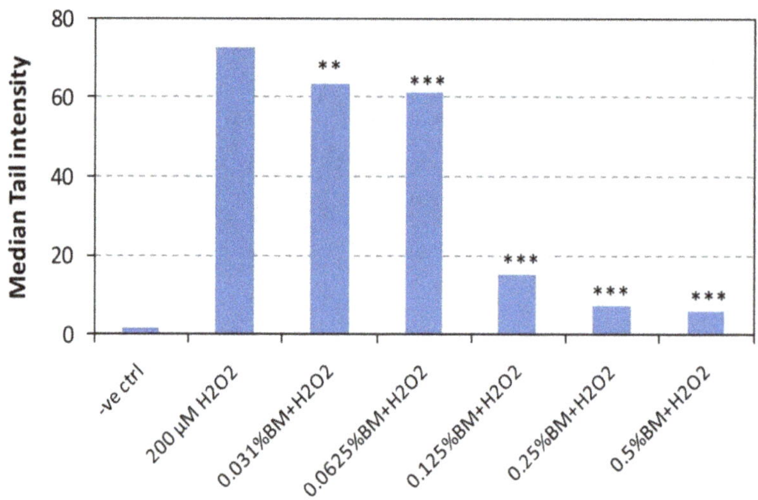

BarleyMax protects DNA in normal colon cells (HT29 cell culture) from oxidative damage by hydrogen peroxide. Two separate experiments are shown. Damage is expressed as a longer DNA tail length in the Comet assay.

DNA damage caused by oxidative stress is one of the earliest events in cancer development. The flavone antioxidants in

BarleyMax (saponarin, lutonarin, and BZ-TMF) provide a biologically credible mechanism for the protection observed here. This was not a pharmaceutical intervention. It was a whole-food system doing what it was designed to do.

What This Research Means, and What It Doesn't

These studies are promising, but preliminary. Cell culture experiments indicate that something biologically interesting is happening, but cancer cells in a laboratory dish behave differently from those in a living person's tumor. Animal studies move closer to biological reality but still do not translate directly to human outcomes. Cancer has been eliminated in animal models many times with agents that proved ineffective or harmful in people. Honest science requires holding that limitation clearly in view.

What the research does establish is that barley grass juice contains compounds, particularly saponarin, lutonarin, and BZ-TMF, that interact with cancer-related biological processes in multiple ways: slowing cell proliferation, promoting cancer cell death, protecting DNA from oxidative damage, and enhancing the immune responses that identify abnormal cells. These are not trivial observations. They are consistent across multiple independent research groups, multiple cancer cell types, and multiple experimental models.

For someone facing a cancer diagnosis or wanting to reduce their long-term cancer risk, barley grass juice powder is a reasonable addition to a serious, comprehensive health strategy. That strategy should include a whole-foods plant-based diet, regular physical activity, restorative sleep, active stress management, and attention to emotional and spiritual well-being. It should involve qualified medical care and honest conversations with practitioners who respect both conventional and natural approaches.

God designed the body with a remarkable capacity for healing. He also designed plants with compounds that support healing in ways we are still discovering. Barley grass juice is one piece of a much larger picture, and in that context, it fills an important role.

Chapter 8

INFLAMMATION, AUTOIMMUNE CONDITIONS, AND TISSUE REPAIR: TRANSLATING EXPERIMENTAL EVIDENCE

Inflammation is the common thread running through most chronic diseases. It underlies rheumatoid arthritis, inflammatory bowel disease, liver injury, and slow wound healing. It accelerates cardiovascular damage, contributes to metabolic dysfunction, and creates the cellular environment in which cancer finds its footing. Understanding how barley grass juice interacts with inflammatory processes is, therefore, not a narrow question. It is central to understanding why this plant system affects so many different conditions.

Research on barley grass juice and inflammation spans cell cultures, animal models, and a single important human trial. Taken together, it points toward a consistent picture: barley grass juice does not suppress inflammation the way a pharmaceutical drug does, by blocking a single pathway regardless of context. Instead, it appears to modulate inflammatory processes, supporting the body's own resolution mechanisms while protecting tissues from oxidative damage.

Suppressing Inflammation at the Cellular Level: The Survival Study

One of the most striking demonstrations of barley grass juice's anti-inflammatory potential comes from a 2013 study by Choi and colleagues, published in *Pharmaceutical Biology*. The researchers tested a methanol extract from barley aerial parts, including leaves similar to those used in barley grass juice, in both cell cultures and animal models exposed to lipopolysaccharide (LPS).

LPS is a bacterial toxin that triggers intense, system-wide inflammation, mimicking the conditions of sepsis. It is one of the most severe inflammatory challenges used in research precisely because it pushes the body's inflammatory response to life-threatening extremes.

In cell cultures, the barley extract significantly reduced inflammatory responses by lowering levels of pro-inflammatory molecules, including nitric oxide and cytokines, the chemical messengers that drive and amplify inflammatory cascades. But the animal experiment produced the most compelling result.

Mice injected with LPS and given no treatment had a survival rate of only 20%. Mice pretreated with barley grass extract survived at an 80% rate.

That fourfold difference in survival under extreme inflammatory conditions is not a subtle finding. It demonstrates that the anti-inflammatory compounds in barley grass extract can protect an organism from inflammation-driven damage at a fundamental level, not merely reducing discomfort, but preserving life under severe physiological stress.

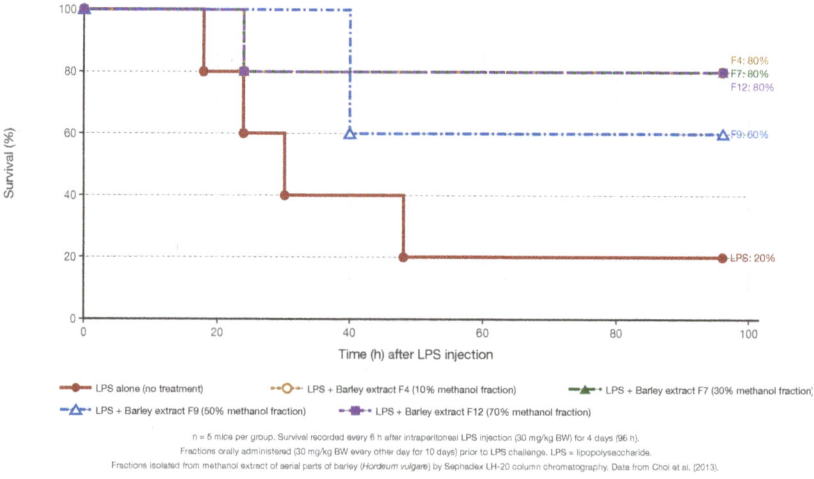

Barley extract prevents death in mice injected with LPS. Data from Choi et al (2013).

The Antioxidant Foundation: Saponarin, Lutonarin, and Vitamin E

Understanding why barley grass juice modulates inflammation so effectively requires returning to its flavone profile. A 2012 study by Kamiyama and Shibamoto, published in the *Journal of Agricultural and Food Chemistry*, examined the flavonoids present in young green barley leaves and measured their antioxidant activity across multiple test systems.

The study confirmed the presence of saponarin and lutonarin as the dominant flavonoids, consistent with the Markham and Mitchell identification discussed in Chapter 3. What it added was a direct measure of their potency: the antioxidant activity of these compounds was comparable to that of vitamin E (alpha-tocopherol) across several assay systems. Vitamin E is one of the most recognized and studied fat-soluble antioxidants in human nutrition. Finding comparable activity in the water-soluble flavones of barley grass juice is a meaningful benchmark.

This distinction between water-soluble and fat-soluble antioxidants is worth noting. Oxidative damage occurs in both the watery interior of cells and in their lipid-rich membranes. A comprehensive antioxidant defense needs to cover both environments. The flavones in barley grass juice, being water-soluble, operate in regions where vitamin E cannot reach, while vitamin E protects the lipid-rich areas where barley flavones are less active. They are complementary rather than redundant, another example of the synergy principle that runs throughout this book.

Inside the Inflammatory Switch: Saponarin, Lutonarin, and NF-κB

Understanding *why* barley grass juice consistently modulates inflammation requires knowing what its two dominant flavones actually do inside an inflamed cell. Two studies from South Korea's National Institute of Crop Science, one published in 2014, one in 2021, answer that question with unusual precision.

The target is a protein complex called NF-κB. Think of it as the master switch for the body's inflammatory response. Under normal conditions, NF-κB remains dormant in the cell's cytoplasm. When a threat is detected, such as a bacterial toxin, an injury signal, or an oxidative insult, NF-κB is released, moves into the cell nucleus, and activates a cascade of genes that drive the production of inflammatory molecules. It is one of the most central control points in the entire inflammatory system, which is why it is also one of the most studied targets in pharmaceutical research on inflammation.

In 2014, Seo and colleagues isolated saponarin from barley sprouts and measured its concentration at approximately 1,143 milligrams per 100 grams of dried sprouts, accounting for 72 percent of the total polyphenol content. They then exposed LPS-activated macrophages to saponarin and measured changes in NF-κB activity. The results were clear. Saponarin suppressed NF-κB activation in a dose-dependent manner by reducing its DNA-binding activity, blocking its entry into the cell nucleus, and decreasing the expression of inflammatory mediators, including IL-

6 and COX-2. Saponarin also inhibited two additional inflammatory signaling pathways, ERK and p38 kinases, adding a second and third layer of suppression on top of the NF-κB effect.

To investigate the mechanism, the researchers used molecular docking simulation, a computational technique that predicts how two molecules physically fit together. Saponarin was found to insert directly into the DNA-binding site of p65, the active component of the NF-κB complex. By occupying that position, saponarin physically prevents NF-κB from binding to DNA and activating its inflammatory targets. It is not a vague or indirect dampening of inflammation. It is a specific molecular interaction at one of the most consequential nodes in the inflammatory system.

In 2021, Yang and colleagues from the same research group returned with an investigation into lutonarin, the second-most abundant flavone in barley seedlings. Lutonarin was present at approximately 1,037 milligrams per 100 grams, only slightly less abundant than saponarin, and its anti-inflammatory activity had not yet been studied. The results closely paralleled those of Seo and colleagues for saponarin. Lutonarin suppressed NF-κB signaling through the same essential mechanism, inhibiting the activation and nuclear movement of its active component, reducing downstream production of the inflammatory cytokines IL-6 and TNF-alpha, and suppressing COX-2 and inducible nitric oxide synthase. Neither compound was toxic to macrophages up to 150 micromolar, a concentration well above the threshold required to demonstrate anti-inflammatory activity.

Taken together, these studies move barley grass juice's anti-inflammatory activity from observation to a mechanistic understanding. The question is no longer just whether these compounds reduce inflammation. There is now a molecular-level answer to how, and the target is one of the most important control points in the entire inflammatory system.

Rheumatoid Arthritis: Modulating an Overactive Immune Response

NF-κB is also a central driver of the inflammation that characterizes rheumatoid arthritis, which makes the next piece of evidence particularly coherent. Rheumatoid arthritis presents a specific inflammatory challenge. Unlike acute inflammation, which resolves once its trigger is removed, the inflammation of rheumatoid arthritis is driven by an immune system that has turned against the body's own joint tissue. Managing it requires modulating immune activity without shutting it down entirely, a delicate balance that pharmaceutical drugs often struggle to achieve without significant side effects.

A 1998 study by Cremer and colleagues, published in the *Romanian Archives of Microbiology and Immunology,* examined the effects of a purified green barley extract on cells taken directly from patients with rheumatoid arthritis. The extract reduced the release of tumor necrosis factor-alpha (TNF-alpha) and reactive oxygen species from these specialized immune cells.

TNF-alpha is one of the central drivers of joint inflammation in rheumatoid arthritis. It is the target of some of the most expensive and widely used pharmaceutical treatments for the condition. The finding that a green barley extract could reduce TNF-alpha release from actual patient cells, rather than just from a general cell line, gives this result particular clinical relevance. It suggests that the extract was interacting with the specific immune dysfunction present in rheumatoid arthritis, rather than merely producing a generalized anti-inflammatory effect.

Inflammatory Bowel Disease: Evidence from Animal Studies

The gastrointestinal tract is one of the most inflammation-prone environments in the body. Conditions like ulcerative colitis involve chronic inflammatory cycles that damage the intestinal lining, impair nutrient absorption, and generate systemic inflammatory signals that affect the entire body.

A 2022 study by Feng and colleagues at China Agricultural University, published in *Nutrients*, examined the effects of barley leaf powder in a mouse model of bacterial colitis. Mice supplemented with barley leaf before infection showed significantly better outcomes than untreated controls, reduced disease severity, less colon damage, lower levels of pro-inflammatory cytokines, including TNF-α and IL-1β, preservation of the intestinal mucosal lining, and lower pathogen burden in feces and organs. Barley leaf also increased beneficial Lactobacillus while reducing harmful Proteobacteria, suggesting a prebiotic-like effect alongside its anti-inflammatory activity.

Notably, the benefit was primarily preventive rather than therapeutic. Mice supplemented before infection fared far better than those supplemented after infection had already begun. This is consistent with the broader principle running through this book: whole-food plant compounds build biological resilience over time rather than acting as acute interventions. It is worth noting that this study used dried whole leaf powder rather than juice powder, so it reflects the contribution of the full barley leaf profile, including dietary fiber and the flavone compounds.

It is also worth noting that mice are somewhat more capable than humans of extracting nutrition from intact plant material, though far less so than true herbivores. The benefits observed here with whole leaf powder, therefore, likely represent a conservative floor rather than the ceiling of what a juice powder, delivering the active compounds in fully bioavailable form, would be expected to achieve.

Wheat Grass Juice for Ulcerative Colitis in People

The most important human evidence in this area comes from a 2002 randomized, double-blind, placebo-controlled trial by Ben-Arye and colleagues, published in the *Scandinavian Journal of Gastroenterology*. This study used wheatgrass juice, a close botanical and phytochemical relative of barley grass, in patients with active distal ulcerative colitis. Participants consumed either 100 ml of wheatgrass juice daily or a placebo for one month.

The results were clinically meaningful. Patients in the wheatgrass group experienced significant reductions in disease activity, including decreased rectal bleeding and abdominal pain, compared with the placebo group.

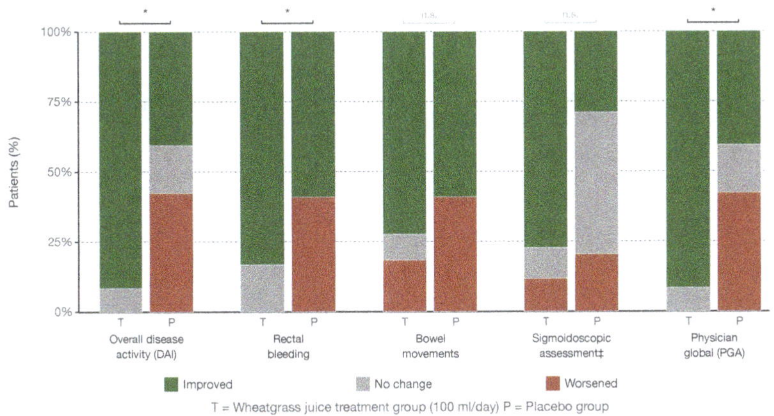

Figure 8.2 Wheat grass juice improves disease activity index in people with active ulcerative colitis. Data from Ben-Arye et al (2002). * = statistically significant difference between groups, p < 0.05; n.s. = not significant; ‡ Sigmoidoscopic data: n = 9 treatment, n = 10 placebo; all others n = 11 treatment, n = 12 placebo. DAI = Disease Activity Index; PGA = Physician Global Assessment.

It is worth noting that the researchers were actually working with tray-grown wheat grass. As described in Chapter 4, tray-grown cereal grass, harvested young from an indoor substrate rather than grown to maturity in open fields, produces a nutritionally inferior product compared to field-grown grass. The Ben-Arye protocol used exactly this: wheat seeds grown indoors on a soil-and-compost substrate in indirect sunlight, harvested at a height of 20 cm. By the standards established in Chapter 4, this is not the strongest possible starting material.

Even so, they got great results. The positive outcomes they saw were more striking, not less, because of this. They obtained meaningful clinical benefits in an active inflammatory disease, achieved with a product that falls short of what field-grown cereal grass or a quality juice powder would deliver. This result deserves serious attention. Of course, it raises the question that can't really be answered here: how much better would the outcomes have been if they had used a more potent source of wheatgrass juice?

This study matters because it is one of the few pieces of human evidence in the cereal grass research record. It demonstrates that cereal grass juice can produce measurable benefits in people with active inflammatory conditions, not just in animal models. Given the strong similarities in flavone profiles and antioxidant activity between wheatgrass and barley grass juice, these findings provide supportive human evidence consistent with the mechanisms observed in barley grass research.

Liver Protection: Guarding a Critical Organ

The liver is the body's primary metabolic processing center and one of the organs most vulnerable to inflammatory damage. A 2017 study by Nepali and colleagues, published in *Phytotherapy Research*, examined a polysaccharide derived from wheatgrass in mice with LPS-induced liver injury, the same bacterial toxin used in the Choi survival study.

The wheatgrass-derived polysaccharide reduced inflammation, oxidative stress, and cell death in liver tissue, protecting it from the damage that LPS exposure would otherwise cause. Polysaccharides are a class of compounds found in both wheatgrass and barley grass, and their presence alongside the flavone profile adds another dimension to the anti-inflammatory activity of cereal grass juice.

For anyone dealing with liver stress, whether from metabolic disease, environmental exposure, or pharmaceutical burden, these findings suggest that the protective compounds in barley grass juice operate across multiple organ systems, not just the gut or the joints.

Wound Healing: When Barley Grass Juice Meets Living Tissue

A 2020 study by Panthi and colleagues in Kathmandu, Nepal, explored the bioactive properties of barley grass extracts and found that the extracts were rich in phenolic and flavonoid content, contributing to strong antioxidant activity. The study also showed that barley grass could stabilize red blood cell membranes, a meaningful indicator of anti-inflammatory capacity, since membrane fragility under oxidative stress is a hallmark of systemic inflammation.

These findings set the stage for a particularly revealing study of wound healing. In 2019, Karbarz and colleagues at the University of Rzeszów in Poland published research examining the effects of freshly squeezed cereal grass juices, including barley grass, on wound healing using an in vitro scratch assay. In this model, a deliberate scratch is made across a layer of cells, and researchers measure how quickly the gap closes.

In normal fibroblasts, the healthy connective tissue cells responsible for wound repair, barley grass juice promoted wound healing through a mechanism researchers described as hormetic. At low doses, the juice stimulated adaptive responses through cellular signaling pathways that enhance antioxidant defenses and accelerate tissue repair. The cells responded to barley grass juice the way living tissue responds to a beneficial challenge: by becoming stronger and more capable.

For people with diabetes, this finding carries particular weight. Slow wound healing is one of the most serious and debilitating complications of poorly controlled blood sugar. High glucose levels impair fibroblast function, slowing the repair process that healthy tissue performs automatically. The ability of barley grass juice to promote healing in normal fibroblasts points to a potential benefit that aligns directly with the metabolic research discussed in Chapter 5.

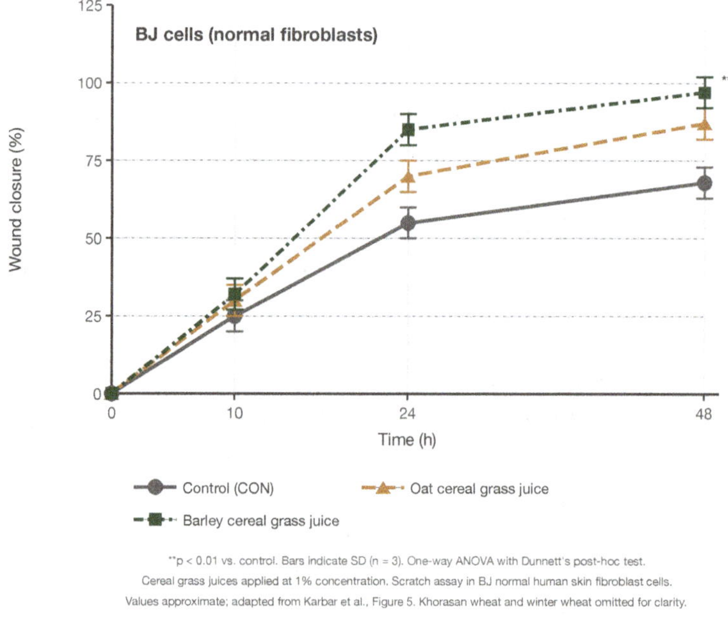

Figure 8.3 Barley grass juice speeds up wound healing in normal fibroblast cells. Data from Karbarz et al (2025).

A Bridge to Cancer: The Dual Action of Barley Grass Juice

What makes the Karbarz study especially remarkable is what happened when the same barley grass juice was applied to cancerous fibroblasts, specifically the ES-2 cancer cell line, rather than healthy ones.

The response was the opposite.

In cancer cells, barley grass juice increased reactive oxygen species and reactive nitrogen species, leading to DNA damage, cell cycle arrest, and impaired wound healing. The same juice that supported and accelerated repair in healthy tissue actively disrupted the growth and repair mechanisms of cancerous tissue.

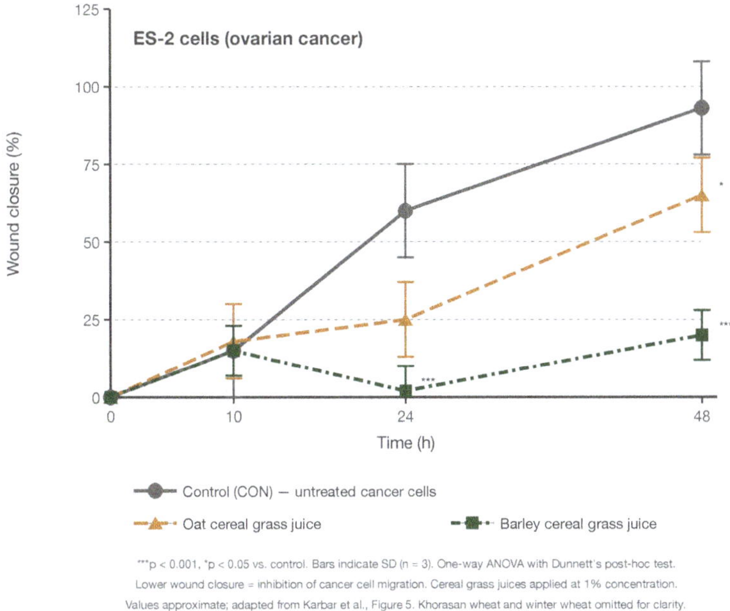

Figure 8.4 Barley grass juice inhibits wound healing in ovarian cancer cells. Data from Karbarz et al (2025).

This dual action (supporting healthy cells while inhibiting cancerous ones) is not what you would expect from a pharmaceutical compound, which typically exerts the same effect on every cell it encounters regardless of that cell's biological status. It is, however, exactly what you might expect from a whole-food plant compound shaped by an infinitely wise and benevolent Creator.

It connects directly to the cancer research examined in Chapter 7, where barley grass extracts consistently spared normal cells while targeting cancer cell lines. The Karbarz wound-healing study provides a mechanistic window into why barley grass juice appears to interact with the biological context of each cell it encounters, supporting normal function while simultaneously disrupting abnormal function.

God's design in the plant kingdom reveals itself in details like this, not a blunt instrument, but a biologically intelligent system that distinguishes between what needs to be supported and what needs to be challenged.

What the Inflammation Research Tells Us

Across cell cultures, animal models, and human evidence, the research on barley grass juice and inflammation tells a consistent story. The active compounds (saponarin, lutonarin, and the broader phytochemical system of the juice) modulate inflammatory pathways, protect tissues from oxidative damage, support the gut lining, defend the liver, and promote tissue repair in ways that pharmaceutical interventions rarely achieve without collateral damage.

None of this research replaces medical treatment for serious inflammatory conditions. Rheumatoid arthritis, ulcerative colitis, and chronic liver disease require professional care and, in many cases, pharmaceutical management. But the evidence suggests that barley grass juice powder can play a meaningful supportive role, working with the body's own resolution mechanisms rather than overriding them.

That is a distinction worth understanding. And it is one that runs through every chapter of this book.

Chapter 9

JUICE POWDER VS. WHOLE-LEAF GRASS POWDER: WHY THIS CHOICE MATTERS TO YOU

Walk into any health food store or browse online supplement retailers, and you will find dozens of products labeled "barley grass." They come in similar green packaging, carry similar health claims, and often sell at similar price points. It would be reasonable to assume they are essentially the same product.

They are not.

The difference between barley grass juice powder and barley grass whole-leaf powder is not a minor technical distinction. It is the difference between extracting what the plant contains and grinding up the plant itself. Understanding this distinction is one of the most practically important things you can take away from this book, because choosing the wrong form means the compounds discussed in every previous chapter may never reach your cells at all.

A Familiar Analogy

Most people have tasted both grape juice and raisins. They come from the same fruit, but their experiences and nutritional profiles are entirely different. Grape juice delivers the water-soluble compounds of the grape in a form that is immediately accessible. Raisins deliver fiber, concentrated sugars, and whatever survives the drying of the whole fruit. Neither is wrong for every purpose, but they are not interchangeable if what you want is the juice.

The same logic applies to barley grass. Barley grass juice powder is made by first extracting the juice from young barley grass, then carefully drying only the juice fraction. The fiber is removed. What remains is a concentrated powder of the water-soluble compounds the plant produced: the flavones, the enzymes, the antioxidants, the phytochemicals that researchers have been studying for decades.

Barley grass whole-leaf powder is made differently. The grass is dried and then ground into fine particles. The fiber stays. The intact plant cells stay. Everything is present on paper, and a nutritional analysis will show vitamins, minerals, and phytochemicals are present. But the critical question is not what is present, but what is accessible.

The Problem with Whole-Leaf Powder

When you eat whole plant foods, your teeth do the first and most important work. Chewing breaks open plant cells, releasing their nutrients. Your digestive system handles the rest. But when whole-leaf barley grass powder is stirred into a glass of water and swallowed, there is no chewing. The particles are already small, but small is not the same as broken open at the cellular level.

Human digestion cannot break down cellulose, hemicellulose, and pectin, the structural components of plant cell walls. We do not have the enzymes for it. Only the nutrients that are actually extracted from intact plant cells become available to your body. Everything still locked inside the cell wall passes through largely unused.

This is why whole-leaf barley grass powder is, in practical terms, expensive fiber. The nutrients show up in the analysis. They do not reliably show up in your bloodstream.

Hay will sustain a cow through the winter because cows have the digestive architecture to extract nutrition from intact grass. We do not. We need the juice.

What Juice Powder Actually Delivers

Barley grass juice powder solves this problem at the source. By extracting the juice before drying, the processing step that matters most, releasing the water-soluble compounds from the plant cells, has already been done. When you mix juice powder into water and drink it, the nutrients are not locked inside anything. They are immediately available for absorption.

This is why the compounds discussed throughout this book (saponarin, lutonarin, BZ-TMF, the antioxidant enzyme systems) are most strongly associated with barley grass juice research rather than whole-leaf powder research. These are water-soluble compounds. They are concentrated in the juice fraction. Grinding up the whole leaf does not concentrate them. It dilutes them within a matrix of indigestible fiber.

The difference is not subtle. In research comparing the two forms, juice powder consistently outperforms whole-leaf powder in biological activity measures. The 2019 Lublin study on colon cancer cells, discussed in Chapter 7, explicitly noted that dehydrated juice powder was a more effective anti-proliferative agent than dried whole-leaf powder, a finding that reflects the same principle operating at the cellular level.

How the Best Barley Grass Juice Powders Are Made

Not all juice powders are made equally. The best producers share a set of practices that distinguish genuinely high-quality processing from shortcuts that compromise the final product. Understanding what that process looks like gives you a benchmark for evaluating any product you consider.

In the best practices, barley is sown in fields enriched through regenerative farming principles. Mineral-rich water supports the plant's nutrient uptake from the soil. The grass grows during the cooler spring and fall seasons, when slower growth allows the plant to accumulate complex antioxidants and phytochemicals that protect it and, in turn, those who consume it.

The grass is harvested at the peak of its nutritional density, with none of it touching the ground. After transport from the field, it is washed, juiced, and quickly chilled. The chilled juice is then dried at the lowest possible temperature, low enough to preserve enzyme activity, in a low-oxygen environment that protects the partially-dried particles from oxidative damage during dehydration. The dried powder is stored cold until bottling and shipping.

The result is a product that smells and tastes like fresh-cut grass, because it essentially is. The vibrancy, the enzymatic life, and the phytochemical complexity of the fresh juice are captured in a stable, convenient powder form. No additives. No carriers. No preservatives. Just the dehydrated juice of young organic barley grass, ready to be mixed into water or a smoothie and absorbed by a body that recognizes it as food.

Enzymes as a Window into Quality

One of the most reliable ways to distinguish a genuinely high-quality barley grass juice powder from a compromised one is enzymatic activity.

As discussed in Chapter 4, enzymes are fragile. They are among the first casualties of aggressive heat processing, prolonged air exposure, or rough handling. If a barley grass juice powder retains measurable enzyme activity, it tells you something important: the processing was gentle enough that the most vulnerable components of the juice survived. If enzyme activity is absent or negligible, it is reasonable to ask what else did not survive.

Whole-leaf barley grass powders, because they require more heat and time to dry intact plant material than extracted juice, consistently show lower enzyme activity than juice powders. Independent testing across multiple commercially available products has clearly confirmed this pattern. Juice powders cluster at the top of the enzyme activity rankings, while whole-leaf powders fall to the bottom, many showing almost no detectable activity at all.

We will examine that testing data in detail in Chapter 10, where specific products are compared and the results are presented directly. For now, the practical takeaway is this: enzymatic activity is not just a measure of one nutrient. It is a proxy for the product's overall biological integrity. A product with robust enzymatic activity has been handled with care to preserve everything else. A product with none has not.

The Bottom Line

Barley grass juice powder and whole-leaf barley grass powder share the same name and color. Beyond that, they are fundamentally different products with fundamentally different biological profiles.

If your goal is fiber, whole-leaf powder may be useful. If your goal is the flavones, enzymes, antioxidants, and phytochemicals that the research in this book describes (the compounds that protect DNA, modulate inflammation, support metabolic health, and strengthen immune function), then juice powder is the only form that reliably delivers them.

This is not a marketing distinction. It is a biochemical one. And it is one that every person choosing a barley grass product deserves to understand. Chapter 10 examines how to verify that what is on the label actually reflects what survives the processing, and gives you the tools to evaluate any barley grass product yourself.

Chapter 10

ENZYMES, CHLOROPHYLL, AND THE WATER TEST: WHAT TESTING ACTUALLY REVEALS

By this point in the book, you understand that barley grass juice powder is not simply a green supplement. It is a living system, captured at a specific moment in a plant's development and preserved through careful handling. The question that naturally follows is a practical one: how do you know whether the product you are buying actually reflects that care, or whether it is a nutritionally compromised powder dressed up in green packaging?

The answer is testing. And as it turns out, there are multiple ways to evaluate what survived the journey from field to jar; some methods require a laboratory, and at least one requires nothing more than a glass of water.

What Independent Testing Actually Looks Like

Before presenting the test results, it is worth explaining how they came to exist, because the story of their development is itself evidence of something important.

When I began working as a research scientist in the field of raw food nutrition in the late 1990s, one of my first priorities was a deceptively simple question: how do you scientifically prove that a food has not been cooked? The value of living, enzymatically active food was central to everything I was investigating, but there was no established method for measuring it consistently across different products. I needed a reliable quality signal. I needed something fragile enough to be destroyed by heat, sensitive enough to distinguish between products processed at different temperatures, and sufficiently measurable to yield quantitative results.

Enzyme testing turned out to be the answer. Enzymes are among the first casualties of heat and oxidation. A food that retains robust enzymatic activity has been processed gently enough for its most vulnerable components to survive. A food without measurable enzyme activity has not. Over time, I settled on a six-enzyme panel to measure the activities of beta-galactosidase, beta-glucosidase, alpha-mannosidase, acid phosphatase, leucine aminopeptidase, and N-acetyl-beta-D-glucosaminidase. These enzymes were chosen because they were easy to monitor with commercially available substrates, were naturally present in sufficient quantities in plants, and the assays were readily adaptable for rapid screening. I designed this panel of enzymes to assess biological vitality across raw food products, including barley grass juice powders.

Over more than two decades, I applied this panel to every significant barley grass product that came to market, tracking quality as the field evolved and new products appeared. The testing was comparative and systematic: all products were tested simultaneously using the same methods under the same conditions. Around 2015, I purchased essentially every commercially available barley grass product (juice powders from a wide variety of brands and all whole-leaf powders) and ran the full panel across them simultaneously. The results are reflected in the ranking table in this chapter.

What Blind Testing Revealed

The most scientifically meaningful findings from this work did not come from the planned comparative studies. They came from something more rigorous: repeated, unplanned blind testing that consistently pointed toward the same conclusion.

The first encounter was almost accidental. A sample of barley grass juice powder had arrived at the laboratory from a producer we were not yet familiar with. It had been sitting in a corner, unexamined, when I ran it through the enzyme panel as part of a routine comparison. The numbers stopped me. The enzymatic activity was higher than anything I had tested up to that point. We requested fresh samples. They were better still.

Only after the testing was complete did I investigate the source. The producer turned out to be the supplier behind what became the highest-ranked product in our comparative analysis.

That alone would have been a strong data point. What made it compelling was that it happened again. And then again.

On a separate occasion, I was evaluating a product from Terrasoul, a brand I was not previously familiar with, as part of a routine quality check. The enzyme activity was strikingly similar to the top-ranked product in our panel. My first thought was that a second producer had achieved the same quality standard. After completing the analysis, I inquired about the source of their powder.

It came from the same producer.

A third incident followed the same pattern. A product from Synergy Laboratories showed enzyme activity at the same elevated level. Same question, same answer: same producer.

In three separate instances, across different brands, purchased at different times, I found enzymatic activity high enough to be remarkable, and in each case, investigation after the fact revealed the same source. I was not looking for confirmation of a hypothesis. I was running routine tests and finding a result I did not expect. The convergence was not something I arranged. It was something I kept discovering.

That is what independent blind testing looks like in practice. Not a designed experiment with pre-registered hypotheses, but repeated, unplanned encounters with the same finding. This kind of blinded testing is the scientific pattern that rigorously defends against the accusation of confirmation bias. When you keep finding the same answer without looking for it, the answer is worth taking seriously.

Enzyme Testing: The Most Sensitive Quality Indicator

The six-enzyme panel applied across commercially available barley grass products divided the market into four recognizable tiers. The pattern was unambiguous.

The top tier consisted of genuine juice powders processed with rigorous low-temperature, low-oxygen methods. These products showed robust enzyme activity across multiple assays, confirming that their processing preserved the biological integrity of the original juice. Among currently available products, BarleyMax, a premium barley grass juice powder produced by Hallelujah Diet, ranked at the top. Its position in the rankings was not assumed or claimed. It was the result of the same blind testing process described above: a product found to perform at the highest level before its source was identified.

The second tier is where the picture becomes more nuanced and more instructive. Several well-known and widely sold juice powder products fell into this range, including Green Magma, Barley Life from AIM International, Barley Grass Juice from NOW Foods, Barley Grass Juice Powder from VitaCost, and BarleyGreen from YH International. These are products with real market presence and genuine name recognition. Some have been industry standards for years. Yet their enzyme activity tells a different story from their labels. The reduction in enzymatic activity across these products indicates that heat was applied during processing, enough to measurably compromise the biological activity of the juice, even if the products retain the juice powder form. Being a juice powder is a necessary condition for quality. It is not, by itself, a sufficient one.

The third tier has only a couple of products that are substantially lower than the second tier, but they're not as bad as the bottom tier. There's still some enzyme activity in these products.

Product	% Rank β-galacto-sidase; 100% = 13.1 U/100g	% Rank β-gluco-sidase; 100% = 22.1 U/100g	% Rank α-manno-sidase; 100% = 223 U/100g	% Rank Acid Phosphatase; 100% = 97.1 U/g	% Rank Leu Amino-peptidase; 100% = 139.5 U/100g	% Rank N-acetyl β-D-glucos-aminidase; 100% = 95.6 U/100g	Average Rank %	RANK
Raw Green Grass, from Juvo	46.5%	100.0%	100.0%	100.0%	62.6%	47.8%	76.2%	1
BarleyMax	68.8%	34.9%	71.9%	42.4%	86.0%	93.9%	66.3%	2
BarleyMax AF	100.0%	27.2%	70.1%	30.3%	81.8%	87.2%	66.1%	3
Just Barley, from Pure Planet	72.6%	37.9%	74.7%	35.3%	68.5%	100.0%	64.8%	4
BarleyMax Berry	41.5%	9.1%	67.3%	51.1%	100.0%	77.5%	57.8%	5
Barley Grass Powder, from Earth Circle Organics	49.1%	27.1%	63.9%	34.2%	45.4%	80.9%	50.1%	6
Barley Grass Juice Powder, from VitaCost (Earthblends)	61.1%	31.0%	46.0%	18.0%	51.5%	32.7%	40.1%	7
Green Magma, from Green Foods	72.6%	12.4%	35.7%	16.7%	52.6%	41.5%	38.6%	8
Barley Grass juice, from NOW Foods	21.5%	13.9%	40.4%	23.9%	51.9%	71.4%	37.1%	9
BarleyLife Traditional, from AIM, Int'l	69.3%	3.4%	44.4%	23.4%	39.8%	35.1%	35.9%	10
Barley Grass Juice Powder, from VitaCost	46.4%	20.7%	37.4%	20.0%	48.9%	33.0%	34.4%	11
BarleyGreen, from YH Int'l	54.6%	10.4%	38.0%	16.9%	33.0%	28.2%	30.2%	12
Alka Green, from Morter Supplements	16.2%	10.5%	16.7%	0.4%	4.7%	9.5%	9.7%	13
Greener Grasses Alkalizer, Healthforce Nutritionals	31.1%	2.5%	5.3%	3.0%	3.5%	3.4%	8.2%	14
Amazing Trio (Barley Grass, Wheat Grass & Alfalfa)	16.2%	0%	3.7%	0.1%	5.6%	3.5%	4.8%	15
Kyo-Green, from Wakunaga	13.6%	0%	0.3%	0%	6.3%	1.7%	3.7%	16
Barley Grass, from Pines	2.7%	0%	0%	0%	6.3%	3.9%	2.2%	17
Barley Grass, from NOW Foods	0%	0%	0%	0%	7.5%	3.2%	1.8%	18
Barley Power, from Green Supreme	0%	0%	3.6%	0%	3.6%	0.5%	1.3%	19
Wheat Grass, from NOW Foods	0%	0%	0%	0%	5.3%	1.3%	1.1%	20
Barley Powder, from Nature's Way	0%	0%	0%	0%	3.1%	0%	0.5%	21
Barley Grass, from Frontier Natural Products	0	0%	0%	0%	0%	0%	0%	22

Rank % calculated as proportion of the highest-observed value for each enzyme class. Average Rank % = mean across all six enzyme classes.

Figure 10.1 Ranking of barley grass products by score on 6-enzyme panel.

The bottom tier confirmed what Chapter 9 predicted. Whole-leaf barley grass powders, regardless of brand, showed almost no detectable enzyme activity across any of the six assays. Products like Barley Grass from NOW Foods, Barley Power from Green Supreme, Barley Powder from Nature's Way, and Barley Grass from Frontier Natural Products registered at or near zero across the board. The nutrients in these products are present on paper. They are not biologically accessible in any meaningful sense.

It is worth noting that this testing was conducted at a specific point in time, and manufacturers do occasionally reformulate their products. The rankings reflect the products as they existed at the time of testing. What they reveal about the relationship between processing care and enzymatic integrity, however, is unlikely to change, because the underlying reason for the difference is not a formulation choice. It is a fundamental consequence of how each product type is made and how carefully its processing conditions are controlled.

Chlorophyll Degradation: What Color Actually Tells You

Enzyme activity is not the only thing that heat destroys. Chlorophyll, the green pigment responsible for photosynthesis and one of the biologically active compounds in barley grass juice, is also vulnerable to heat and acid exposure.

Most people have witnessed chlorophyll degradation without realizing it. A fresh green bean is a vivid shade of green. Cook it briefly, and it brightens momentarily as trapped air escapes. Cook it too long, and it turns a dull, olive drab color. That color change is not cosmetic. It reflects a specific chemical transformation: the magnesium atom at the center of the chlorophyll molecule has been displaced, converting chlorophyll into a compound called pheophytin.

Pheophytin is not chlorophyll. It does not carry the same biological activity. And its presence in a green powder is a direct indicator that the processing conditions were harsh enough to damage one of the plant's most fundamental molecules.

This transformation can be measured precisely using a ratio called the PQa value, the ratio of light absorbance at 435 nanometers to absorbance at 415 nanometers. Fresh, undamaged chlorophyll produces a PQa value of 1.41. Completely pheophytinized material, where all the chlorophyll has been converted, produces a value of 0.56. Everything in between reflects a degree of degradation proportional to the processing conditions the product experienced.

Food	*N, number of samples*	*PQa, Abs 435 / Abs 415*
Fresh spinach	6	1.25
Frozen spinach	6	1.20
Canned spinach	2	0.59
BarleyMax	8	1.06
Product A	8	0.78
Green pepper	2	1.35
Broccoli (green buds only)	2	1.32
Wheat grass leaf	4	1.40
Wheat grass juice	4	1.32
Lawn grass juice	4	1.27

Figure 10.2 PQa values for common foods, showing amount of chlorophyll damage.

The table tells a clear story. Fresh raw vegetables score high: fresh spinach at 1.25, green pepper at 1.35, broccoli at 1.32. These are foods that have not been exposed to significant heat. Wheat grass leaf scores 1.40, essentially perfect, as you would expect from undried plant material. Wheatgrass juice drops slightly to 1.32, reflecting the modest effect of juicing.

Canned spinach tells the other side of the story. At 0.59, it sits just above the fully pheophytinized threshold of 0.56. Anyone who has seen canned spinach knows exactly what that number looks like, the drab, olive-colored result of high-heat sterilization. The magnesium is gone. The chlorophyll is gone. What remains carries the name but not the biology.

BarleyMax measured at 1.06 across eight samples, indicating some loss of magnesium during processing, as is unavoidable when converting fresh juice into a shelf-stable powder, but retaining the majority of its chlorophyll integrity. A competing product measured in the same analysis, referred to here as Product A, scored 0.78 across eight samples, indicating significantly greater chlorophyll degradation and more severe processing conditions.

The difference between 1.06 and 0.78 is not subtle. It represents a meaningful gap in how gently each product was handled and, by extension, a gap in how much of the juice's broader biological complexity survived into the final product.

The Water Test: Check Barley Grass Quality at Home

Not everyone has access to enzyme assay equipment or a spectrophotometer. But there is a simple, practical test that anyone can perform with nothing more than a glass of water and a few hours of patience, and it reveals more about product quality than most people realize.

Here is how it works. Mix a serving of barley grass powder into a clear glass of water. Stir it well, then set it aside and leave it undisturbed for two to four hours. Come back and observe what has happened.

A high-quality, low-temperature dried juice powder will remain largely in suspension. The water will stay green. Very little will settle to the bottom, and the color throughout the glass will remain consistent. Left even longer, it will not turn brown.

A whole-leaf powder will behave differently. Because it consists largely of dried plant fiber particles, it will settle. The heavier material sinks to the bottom, leaving a separation between the settled solids and the water above.

But the most telling result comes from a heat-processed product, whether juice powder or whole-leaf, that has been dried at high temperatures. These products will often produce brown water. The green color fades or separates, leaving a brownish, watery middle layer that no amount of stirring can permanently correct.

That brown color is pheophytin. It is the visible signature of damaged chlorophyll, the same transformation measured in the laboratory by the PQa ratio, now visible to the naked eye in a glass on your kitchen counter. If your barley grass product turns the water brown, the chlorophyll has been compromised. And if the chlorophyll has been compromised, it is reasonable to ask what else has been as well.

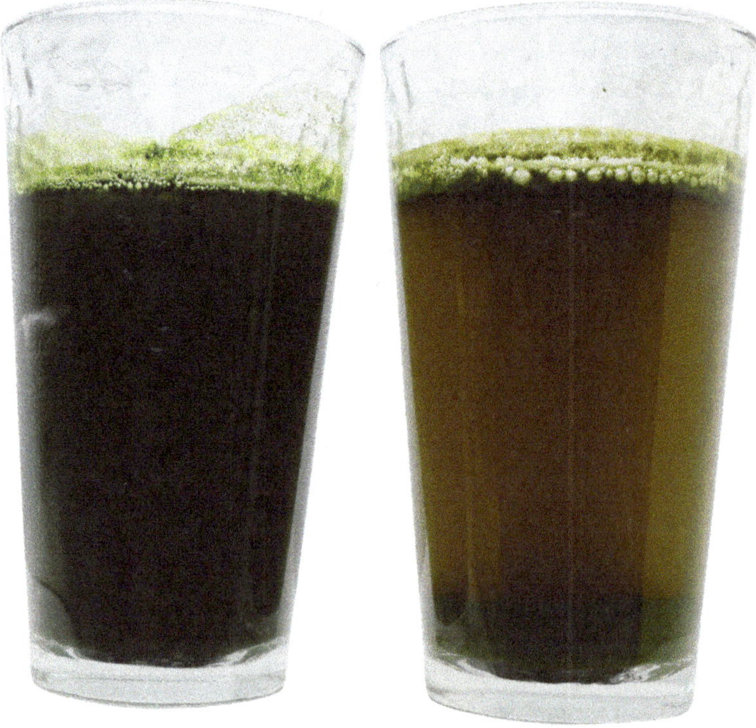

Figure 10.3 Water test with high-quality and medium-quality barley grass juice powder.

This test is qualitative rather than quantitative. It will not tell you exactly how much chlorophyll survived, or give you an enzyme activity number. But it is a meaningful first filter. A product that passes the water test, staying green, staying in suspension, not browning, has at minimum been processed gently enough to preserve its chlorophyll. A product that fails has not.

What These Three Measures Tell You Together

Enzyme activity, chlorophyll integrity, and the water test do not measure the same thing. But they are asking the same question from different angles: did the processing preserve what makes this product biologically valuable, or did it destroy it?

A product that scores well on all three measures (high enzyme activity, a PQa value above 1.0, and water that stays green) has been handled with the care that the research in this book demands. The flavones, the enzymes, the chlorophyll derivatives, the full complement of compounds that interact with human biology in the ways described across the previous eight chapters, are most likely to be present and intact.

A product that fails on these measures may still be green. It may still carry an impressive label. But the biology that justifies those claims has been compromised during processing, before it ever reaches the consumer.

This is not a minor distinction. It is the difference between a product that resembles the biologically active material studied in research and one that merely resembles it in color and name.

Transparency as a Standard

Producers who are confident in their processing will be willing to share their testing data. Enzyme activity results, chlorophyll integrity measurements, and independent quality verification are not proprietary secrets. They are the evidence that separates a serious product from a marketing exercise.

When evaluating any barley grass product, the questions worth asking are straightforward. Is this a juice powder or a whole-leaf powder? What enzyme activity does it retain? Has chlorophyll integrity been measured? Is independent testing data available?

If a producer cannot or will not answer these questions, the water test is always available. It costs nothing, requires no equipment, and tells you something real about what you are holding in your hand.

God designed barley grass to be a living, biologically active food. Preserving that life through processing is both a scientific challenge and a responsibility. The testing described in this chapter exists to verify that the responsibility has been taken seriously and to give consumers the tools to recognize when it has not.

Chapter 11

LIFE COMES FROM LIFE: WHAT THE EVIDENCE MEANS AND HOW TO USE IT

This book began with a simple observation, one that predates modern biochemistry, HPLC analysis, and NMR spectroscopy, and predates every study cited in the preceding chapters. Life comes from life. Living food carries something that processed, degraded, or fragmented food does not. Early researchers felt this intuitively. They called what they observed the grass juice factor, carefully named it, rigorously documented it, and honestly admitted that they could not fully explain it.

Ninety years later, we can explain much more of it. And what the explanation reveals is not simpler than the original observation. It is richer, deeper, and more remarkable.

The Arc of the Evidence

The story that has unfolded across these chapters is not a straight line from discovery to confirmation. It is the kind of story that real science produces: full of wrong turns, careful corrections, and findings that raise as many questions as they answer.

It began with Schnabel and his colleagues in the 1930s, documenting effects in animals that no single identified nutrient could account for. It continued through decades of research that gradually mapped the biochemical landscape of young barley grass, revealing flavones, enzymes, chlorophyll derivatives, and antioxidant systems working together in ways that consistently exceeded what isolated compounds could replicate.

It took a wrong turn in 1992, when careful analytical work misidentified the dominant flavonoid in young barley leaves as a novel compound called 2"-O-GIV. It was corrected in 2003, when Markham and Mitchell did the detective work that established the truth: the dominant compounds were saponarin and lutonarin, well-characterized flavone-C-glycosides with potent antioxidant activity and water solubility, which concentrate in the plant's juice fraction. And it expanded further with the identification of BZ-TMF (a methylated flavone that accounted for a significant proportion of the phytochemicals detected in barley grass powder in one analysis), whose influence on metabolic signaling provided a long-awaited explanation for the glucose-regulating effects observed in diabetic animal models.

Each chapter of this book added a layer to that picture. The metabolic health research in Chapter 5 showed that barley grass compounds act at the level of hepatic glucose regulation and beta-cell preservation, protecting the very insulin-producing tissue that diabetes progressively destroys. The mental health research in Chapter 6 showed flavones and neuroprotective factors interacting with stress signaling in the brain, preserving BDNF and modulating the neurochemical environment in which resilience either holds or collapses. The cancer research in Chapter 7 showed barley grass extracts selectively targeting abnormal cells while leaving healthy ones intact, the same biological intelligence that wound-healing research confirmed from a different angle in Chapter 8. Inflammation research showed a fourfold difference in survival under septic conditions; inhibition of NF-κB signaling by saponarin and lutonarin in LPS-activated macrophages; modulation of TNF-α in rheumatoid arthritis patient cells; and meaningful clinical benefit in human ulcerative colitis patients, even though they received only tray-grown cereal grass juice.

And through it all (every chapter, every study, every mechanism) one principle held constant. The effects came from the whole juice. Not from an extracted flavone. Not from a concentrated isolate.

From the living system, captured at its peak and preserved with sufficient care to remain biologically active when it reached the person drinking it.

What We Don't Yet Know

Honest science requires holding its limitations clearly in view, and this book has tried to do that at every step.

The majority of the research reviewed here was conducted in animals, primarily rats and mice, under experimental conditions that do not directly map onto human disease. Streptozotocin-induced diabetes in a rat is not type 2 diabetes in a person who has lived with metabolic dysfunction for twenty years. Forced swim tests in mice capture something real about stress resilience and neuroprotection, but they are not the same as the lived experience of clinical depression. Cell cultures show biological mechanisms operating in controlled conditions that the complexity of the human body does not replicate.

Human clinical trials on barley grass juice are limited. The Ben-Arye wheatgrass trial in patients with ulcerative colitis is one of the few pieces of rigorous human evidence in the entire cereal grass research record. It is encouraging, but a single trial in a single condition does not constitute a body of human evidence.

What is needed, and what does not yet exist in sufficient quantity, is well-designed human research. Randomized controlled trials examining barley grass juice powder in people with type 2 diabetes, inflammatory bowel disease, metabolic syndrome, and elevated cardiovascular risk. Studies with standardized products, measured doses, and outcomes that matter to patients. We are ready to measure not just biomarkers, but quality of life, disease progression, and long-term health trajectories.

The animal and laboratory evidence reviewed in this book is not preliminary in the dismissive sense. It is mechanistically coherent, consistent across independent research groups, and biologically plausible in ways that justify serious human investigation. But it is not yet the final word. Anyone reading this book deserves to know that, and to hold the findings with appropriate hope rather than false certainty.

Barley Grass Juice in the Larger Picture

The story of barley grass juice is compelling on its own terms. But it is also part of a larger story, one that runs through turmeric and ginger, berberine and ashwagandha, ginseng and maca, and dozens of other well-researched plant compounds that have accumulated meaningful evidence for their effects on human health.

What unites these compounds is not merely that they are natural. It is how they work. They do not operate like pharmaceutical drugs, hitting a single molecular target with maximum force and accepting the collateral damage that comes with it. They interact with biological systems intelligently. They support what needs to be supported, challenge what needs to be disrupted, and do so in ways that distinguish healthy from aberrant tissue with a precision no synthetic compound has yet to replicate.

This is not an accident of chemistry. It is the signature of design. These compounds were shaped to work within living systems because they come from living systems. They are produced by organisms that share, at a fundamental level, the same biochemical language as the bodies that consume them. A Creator who understood biology at this level of depth and integration did not leave His design unfinished. The evidence of that design is visible in every study reviewed in this book: in the selectivity of barley grass flavones for cancer cells over healthy ones, in the dual action that promotes healing in normal fibroblasts while disrupting it in cancerous ones, in the metabolic intelligence of BZ-TMF acting on glucose pathways without inducing hypoglycemia.

And the evidence did not come from one place, or one tradition, or one scientific culture. Researchers in Poland, Egypt, Nepal, Japan, Slovakia, China, and the United States all independently discovered barley grass juice. Their journey was not because a pharmaceutical company funded the investigation, but because people were using it, reporting results, and curious minds around the world followed the evidence. The science in this book is genuinely global, driven not by commercial interest but by the oldest motivation in research: something was happening that needed to be understood. Ordinary people drank barley grass juice and experienced results they could not fully explain. Scientists noticed, investigated, and found mechanisms that confirmed what experience had already suggested. That chain, from human observation to laboratory investigation to biochemical explanation, is how the most trustworthy science gets made. And it is the chain that connects every study in this book to the people whose lives prompted the questions in the first place.

Barley grass juice is one expression of a principle that runs through the entire plant kingdom. Eat close to the way you were designed to eat, choosing whole foods, living foods, foods that retain the biological complexity that processing strips away, and you give your body the biochemical vocabulary it needs to do what it was designed to do: regulate, repair, defend, and heal.

What the Testing Tells You

Understanding the science is one thing. Applying it in practice requires knowing that the product you choose accurately reflects what the research describes. As Chapters 9 and 10 made clear, not all barley grass products are equivalent, and the differences between them are not minor.

A genuine barley grass juice powder, processed at low temperature in a low-oxygen environment and stored cold, retains the enzyme activity, chlorophyll integrity, and phytochemical complexity that make the research relevant to your body. A whole-leaf powder, regardless of how it is marketed, does not deliver these compounds in a bioavailable form. And a heat-processed juice powder, whatever its label claims, has sacrificed the biological integrity that distinguishes a living food from an expensive green powder.

The water test, the PQa chlorophyll ratio, and independent enzyme testing are not academic exercises. They are the tools that connect the science to the product in your hand. Use them.

How to Use Barley Grass Juice Powder

At this point in the book, practical guidance does not require elaborate instruction. The research does not specify a precise human dose. It cannot, given that the evidence base is primarily animal studies with doses that do not translate directly to humans. What it suggests is that consistent daily use of a high-quality juice powder, at whatever amount fits your life and budget, is likely to be more valuable than occasional large doses.

A small daily serving, as little as two grams, delivers compounds that are simply not available in meaningful amounts from any other commonly consumed food. Saponarin and lutonarin do not appear in significant concentrations elsewhere in the typical diet. BZ-TMF is not found in spinach, broccoli, or any standard green vegetable. These compounds are specific to young cereal grass juice, and the only way to get them consistently is to include a high-quality juice powder in your daily routine.

More is not always better, and there is no established optimal dose for humans. What matters more than the amount is the consistency and the quality. Two grams of a genuine low-temperature-dried juice powder every day is worth more than 10 grams of a heat-processed whole-leaf powder taken sporadically.

Mix it into water, into a smoothie, or into whatever daily habit you can sustain without friction. The best dose is the one you actually take.

A Final Word

The grass juice factor was never fully explained by any single discovery. It was gradually illuminated by researchers willing to look closely at something that early science had noticed but could not account for. What they found, over nine decades of investigation, was not one thing. It was a system, a biologically coherent, intelligently designed system of compounds working together in ways that support life at the cellular level.

That system did not assemble itself by accident. It was placed in creation by a God who understood what human bodies would need long before human scientists had the tools to study it. The evidence reviewed in this book is, among other things, a record of those discoveries, of human inquiry gradually catching up to a design that was always already there.

Life comes from life. It always has. The science, at its best, is simply the long process of learning to see what that means.

Success Stories

EDITORIAL NOTE

The testimonies in this chapter were collected by Hallelujah Diet, whose branded barley grass juice powder product is BarleyMax. They are presented here in the contributors' own words, with only light editing for clarity. References to BarleyMax, Hallelujah Acres, and Reverend Malkmus reflect the context in which these experiences occurred and have not been altered. BarleyMax is an example of a premium barley grass juice powder produced through low-temperature processing, the same category of product discussed throughout this book. The experiences described here are consistent with the biological mechanisms reviewed in the preceding chapters, and they are offered in that spirit: not as medical claims, but as human accounts of what became possible when living food was taken seriously.

SUCCESS STORIES

Over the years at Hallelujah Acres, we have received accounts from people who incorporated BarleyMax into their daily routine, sometimes as a first step toward broader health changes, or sometimes as a single addition to an already healthy lifestyle. As I noted in the opening chapter of this book, small changes have a way of building momentum, encouraging people to keep going in their pursuit of health.

It is not always possible to know precisely how much of what someone experiences is due to the barley grass juice powder itself and how much reflects the cumulative effect of other positive changes happening at the same time. It's more important to me to be honest than to make a compelling claim. What I can say is that the people whose stories follow attribute meaningful changes in their health to BarleyMax, and that their experiences are consistent with the biological mechanisms described throughout this book.

These accounts are presented in the contributors' own words, very lightly edited for clarity. They are not intended as medical claims. They are human and pet experiences, offered in the hope that they might encourage others who are still searching.

Disclaimer

The testimonies in this chapter represent individual experiences and are not intended as medical advice or as claims that BarleyMax treats, cures, or prevents any disease or health condition. Individual results vary. The experiences described here have not been independently verified and may reflect the combined effects of multiple lifestyle and dietary changes rather than those of BarleyMax alone. If you are managing a health condition, please consult a qualified healthcare provider before making changes to your diet or supplement routine.

More BarleyMax for Better Sleep Without Drugs

I had been unable to sleep for the past four years without a sleep aide. I had tried everything both natural and pharmaceutical.

I had to sleep and sadly, only the prescription drugs worked. Anyone who can't sleep knows the trap this becomes when only drugs allow you to sleep.

Well recently, I decided to try upping the recommended servings of BarleyMax of two to three servings a day to six and eight servings a day and the "side effect" was that I could sleep and without needing any drugs.

I am so glad to be able to stop the pharmaceuticals. Whatever it was that I was missing and that kept me from sleeping, BarleyMax gave me. What an unexpected and glorious surprise.

Thank you Rev. Malkmus for sharing your story and leading this wonderful Hallelujah Acres Ministry. I am ever grateful.

— Brenda M.

BarleyMax Helped Carla Get Through a Difficult Mission Trip

I just returned from three weeks of mission work in Zambia and the Congo.

I wanted to touch base and give you an idea of the success I had being on the Hallelujah Acres Diet, at least the best I could under the circumstances on this missionary trip.

There were five others on the trip with me who were not on the Hallelujah Diet, and though I was not able to get any fresh veggies or fruits, I faithfully took my BarleyMax (6 teaspoons per day) and even though I out-aged the others by a minimum of 13 years, I ran circles around them and had more energy than any of them. Some of those with me were 22 years younger.

And though I did have to eat some unidentifiable things in the bush villages; I did not experience any illness except some throat and breathing irritation from the constant smoke from fires in the villages that were burning around me 24 hours a day.

I sometimes rode for hours crammed in a small vehicle with 23 other people, mostly natives. I slept on things that most would not consider beds, and we were even arrested by a team claiming we were American terrorists. Fortunately we were able to bargain for our release out of the Congo.

Anyway, to make a long story short, along with BarleyMax and some probiotics I made it through the trip without any illnesses.

— Carla C. - Palm Bay, FL

BarleyMax Helps Infant with Side Effects of Chemo

Our daughter was diagnosed with AML-M7 (Acute Myeloid Leukemia Type M7) last Nov. 23, 2002. She was a week away from her 2nd birthday! She did 6 months of intensive chemotherapy. She relapsed a month later, did 2 rounds of salvage chemo and is now recovering from an amazing cord blood transplant. She is on day plus 11 and she is in the part where her body is en grafting. Her name is Trinity and she is bright, brilliant, and so beautiful.

Enough said, I have used BarleyMax since Dec. of last year and have gone through at least 10, 8.5 oz. tubs of BarleyMax. The results are sooooo phenomenal that I have gotten up to 10 different cancer patients on it, and the energy that my daughter has received from this gift from God is amazing, the effects of chemo are horrendous and have saved my Trinity from mouth sores, mucousitis, swelling, fatigue, diarrhea, and the most significant overall incredible result from the BMax is the energy our daughter has and had during her chemo is once again phenomenal. Doctors and nurses alike are amazed at the energy she possesses.

Many parents are beginning to approach me on what I give our daughter and have told our Oncologist about it. He is Dr. Kirk Schultz, an immunologist/oncologist and does a lot of research and he said that if your company supplies the BarleyMax he would do a research study on its benefits, etc. Please, if anything can be done, hold our oncologist to his word. The news about how this has enables our Trinity to have a decent course of chemo with almost zero side effects needs to be known. One mother that has her daughter on BarleyMax, claims it helps her daughter's hemoglobin, red blood cell counts rise post chemo faster.

— Elaine J.

Nursed Back to Health with BarleyMax, Digestive Enzymes, Probiotics, and Fresh Juice

I was away the entire month of August taking care of my sister who had cancer. The results were fantastic! When I arrived, she was very,

very sick. She had been told on June 28 that she had stage-4 breast cancer, and for the entire month of July had been in and out of the hospital - more in than out. The cancer was spreading very rapidly and she was in a lot of pain. They had already drained 2 gallons of fluid from her stomach twice. The cancer had started in her breast and had spread to her stomach and bones. She was on a puffer for a bad cough, caused by the fluid build up. The doctors had placed her on medication for the cancer in her bones, and had given her one bout of chemo. For the entire month of July, she had not been able to eat or drink hardly anything, had lost 30 pounds, and was having a terrible time keeping anything down.

When I arrived, I started her immediately on BarleyMax the first day. On the second day it was BarleyMax, and I added probiotics and enzymes. On the evening of the second day we got a juicer that our other sister had. On the third day she received BarleyMax, probiotics, enzymes, and carrot juice, along with a little raw food in the evening, which she was able to keep down. By day 4, she felt so much better that she couldn't wait for her lunch. On day 5 she went to church, and was well enough on the 6th day that we were able to go to a hot springs resort for the day. On about the 5th day, I started her on Fiber Cleanse along with BeetMax, as well as the B-12.

Her results were nothing short of miraculous! By the time I came home (after only one month), she was out shopping, helping to make dinner and juice, and told me she did not feel like she had cancer anymore. She had had her stomach pumped out 3 days before I arrived for the second time, but this was not necessary again after I started her on The Hallelujah Diet, along with those supplements. Her cough went away in 3 days, and the pain from the cancer in her ribs went away after a week. It was at this point that she decided on her own to not go for any more chemo and to also stop all her medications. God is so good!

— Health Minister Ellie Stalker of Lake Charles, LA

BarleyMax, Fresh Juices Spur on Good Health

Hi George, I have been juicing and using BarleyMax for several months now and have seen a definite improvement in my general health. I have already gotten off my blood pressure medicine and cholesterol medication, and my hemorrhoids are gone! Hallelujah! I drink at least 24 ounces of carrot juice daily, plus other juices from my Champion Juicer. I eat apples, oranges, and bananas throughout the day, drink BarleyMax three times a day, and eat a large salad in the evening. Plus, I drink plenty of purified water throughout the day. I am serious about getting in better shape. I am 55-years old, and after only a few months on The Hallelujah Diet, feel that I am in great shape. Thanks for all your info, encouraging letters, and interest in others.

 — Phil B.

BarleyMax Helps with MS

Hello! I was diagnosed with Multiple Sclerosis in November 2005. In December 2005 I went on The Hallelujah Diet after going to the Hallelujah Acres Lifestyle Center in Lake Lure North Carolina, which is run by Bev and Chet Cook.

Before adopting The Hallelujah Diet, the doctors told me I must use Interferon, but I decided to go God's way instead. Since adopting The Hallelujah Diet I have been doing great! I walk every morning for one hour, drink vegetable juices and BarleyMax, while eating lots of raw veggies and fruit. I only have thankful thoughts about the diet and wish that everybody could do this wonderful God's Way Diet and Lifestyle.

 — Rocio of Oakton, VA

BarleyMax and Hallelujah Diet Brighten Sara's Outlook as She Regains Hope

I have been depressed since childhood, hospitalized, and diagnosed with chronic severe depression. I tried medication, but it only made me numb. Over the years, I lost interest in almost everything, and believed there was no help or hope for me. I have even been suicidal off and on since I was 16.

After years of depression, I began to believe I wasn't worth killing, because of the hassle, expense, and problems it would cause others. I didn't believe I deserved to be in the Hallelujah Acres Get Healthy class that first night I attended.

But after starting The Hallelujah Diet, and the BarleyMax, and carrot juice, within 2-3 days, the black cloud and obsessive thinking that told me that I was not worth killing had lifted, and life became brighter. It was then that I began to feel that there was hope for a better life and a reason to get healthy. This was so unexpected and my energy has increased greatly, and I know that things will only get better! My husband Paul and I are coming to Health Ministers training in November.

— Sara of North Carolina

BarleyMax Helps with Fibromyalgia Fatigue

My husband and I have been using Barley Green and now Barley Max for approximately 1 1/2 years. My daughter (25) has always been very active, she is a black belt in karate, has her degree in English and teaches High School English and worked out every day.

About 4 years ago she began to be very tired, with joint aches, headaches, etc. Many doctors and many medications later, she was diagnosed with fibromyalgia. The med's just made her a zombie and didn't really help with the pain. I asked her to try the Barley Green. She did and approximately 1 month after beginning to add Barley Green and FiberBlend to her day, she was feeling so much better. She has since been pretty symptom free, even exercising up to 1 hour a day! She ran out of Barley Green and didn't want to ask to use ours, after 2 weeks her fibro symptoms returned! She was so sad, she didn't want to live that way again. I gave her my BarleyMax and it took about a week to restore her to good health again. Needless to say, we won't be out of Barley Max again! Praise the Lord for leading you in this ministry.

— Deana

BarleyMax and Hallelujah Diet Help Extend Life of 87-Year Old Mom

Dear Rev. Malkmus, I wanted to write and share how The Hallelujah Diet has helped my 87-year-old mother. In January 2006 my mom became very ill and ended up in the hospital's emergency room. Her blood pressure was 238/120, she was unable to communicate (possibly as a result of a stroke), had severe peripheral artery disease, was extremely anemic, and they discovered a large tumor on her kidney. The doctor we consulted with that night told us that I needed to call any family members who wanted to see her alive one last time, and that I should tell them to come quickly.

Knowing mom's only hope was The Hallelujah Diet or die, I started bringing carrot juice and BarleyMax to her while in ICU. She started to improve, and when they released her, I brought her to my home and put her completely on The Hallelujah Diet. I also took her off Pepsi, along with white flour products, meat and cheese, and other harmful foods.

Within 3-weeks of starting The Hallelujah Diet, we all noticed she was getting noticeably stronger! However, the pain in her legs from peripheral artery disease was just too intense. The doctors said she only had a 5% blood flow and said she must have bi-pass surgery or lose her leg. Having been on The Hallelujah Diet for only 3-weeks, I knew it wasn't a long enough period of time to correct all the physical problems created by being all those years on the SAD diet, so I felt I had to give the doctors permission to perform the surgery even though the doctors said she might not survive the surgery.

Well, it is now late summer 2006, and it has been 9-months since the doctors told me that my mom wouldn't make it through the night and the doctors don't know what to make of my mom. Her blood pressure is now regularly 120/80, and they have taken her off one of her medications. Her anemia has improved by 75%.

Since August she has been going to her old Bible Study along with other activities. She is doing much better communicating and always has a smile on her face. Thank you Dr. Malkmus, without your wisdom I wouldn't have had the last 9-months with my mother and they have been priceless! Blessings. P.S. I've enclosed a picture of her so that you can see how wonderful she looks.

— Debbie

Barley Grass Juice Powder Leads to Health Transformation

Last spring I asked that you send the book "Back to the Garden" to my daughter and me in Virginia. She was in very poor health, because most of her body systems appeared to be deteriorating.

She started drinking dehydrated barley juice powder and carrot juice. We have just visited her again, and Wow! She looks like our daughter again. Not some stranger. We thank y'all and praise God.

— Anonymous

Her Guinea Pig Thrived on BarleyMax

I have a very different kind of testimony that may be of interest to pet lovers. In July of this year I bought a pair of guinea pigs from a local pet store. They were both young and beautiful. After a few days at home, I noticed that the female was having loud, labored breathing. When I took her to the vet, he told me she had a severe respiratory infection, probably pneumonia, and that there was a good chance she might not make it.

My two options were to take the guinea pig back to the store and demand another one or to keep this one and try to nurse it back to health. The vet and I agreed that the store would probably not do anything to restore the guinea pig's health if I returned it, so I decided to keep it and see what we could do at home. The vet put her on antibiotics that gave her diarrhea and caused her to lose her appetite. Since I drank BarleyMax greens every morning, I decided to save the last sip and feed it each morning to the guinea pig with a syringe. I thought I'd have to force feed it to her, but she absolutely loved the taste! In fact, I couldn't get her to let go of the syringe easily. She was like a baby with a bottle!

I saw her health improve. She even had a severe infestation of mites (which I'm sure she brought with her from the pet store) and had to receive strong injections of medication for that. Once again, she lost her appetite, but the Barley Green nursed her back to health. In conclusion, this frail, sick little guinea pig that nearly died a few months ago is now strong, healthy, large, and expecting!

We've long known that guinea pigs have been used as experimental animals for testing of products and medicines. I put our guinea pig to the test with Barley Green and she passed with flying colors! If it did this much good for a small mammal, can you believe what good it must do for large mammals like ourselves? By the way, instead of buying the pet store junk food for our guinea pigs, they follow a Hallelujah Diet of fresh fruit and vegetables and distilled water every day of their lives and they are thriving because they are eating the foods that God created their bodies to ingest. Interesting, isn't it?

— Carol G. - Sarasota

BarleyMax Helps Cat Regain Strength

Hi George and Olin,

I need to share this with you, as I had sent some information to you earlier which indicated that Alfalfa was poisonous to cats. I wondered if BarleyMax was safe to use in their food.

One of the stray cats we feed was missing for some time, then showed up two weeks ago so sick he couldn't walk a straight line. Just trying to climb the one 6 step to our back door, caused him to fall and lose his balance. He was very thin, couldn't seem to meow, and it didn't look like he was long for this world. I prayed over him, and decided to try BarleyMax in his food. I didn't think he could get any worse without dying and felt it was his only chance to survive.

Each morning, noon, and evening I gave him small servings of a good quality canned cat food with about 1/8 tsp. of BarleyMax greens. He couldn't eat much food at one setting, but he ate every bite, and within two days I could see an improvement. Today, two weeks later, he appears to be 98% back to his normal healthy condition. His weight is back to normal. He walks soundly with a spring back in his step, meows with excitement again, is able to jump up onto a 29" table without losing his balance, and seems happy again.

What a difference in such a short time! This answers the Alfalfa question for me. At least in the form it takes in BarleyMax. It surely was not poisonous to my cat! Thanks for the good work you all do! God bless you richly!

— Francine T.

BarleyMax Helps Extend Life of Family Pet

We had a Samoyed, who at 11-1/2 years old, we got a diagnosis from our vet that he had liver cancer. The prognosis was that he would live 1 - 3 months at best.

She prescribed pain medication as needed. Niki did not seem to be in pain at the time, so we held off on starting pain medication, but I did add barley max to his diet, and included some raw vegetables in his food.

He lived another 1-1/2 years, during which time he thoroughly enjoyed his walks and showed no signs of real illness or pain til the last month of his life.

The vet was very amazed at how well he was doing, and said to just keep doing whatever we were doing as it was obviously working.

We have had a niece and friends who's pets also developed different types of cancers, although we felt we were feeding high quality food without additives, etc.

I believe that the environment, lawn chemicals, and insecticides that are so heavily used everywhere now, contributes to our pets illnesses.

Niki was not cured of the liver cancer, but I am certain that the addition of the barley max to his diet gave us more than an extra year with our precious Niki, and gave him a quality of life during that time that he would not have had. A samoyed's life expectancy is around 13 to 14 years, so thanks to Hallelujah Acres, Niki lived out that time with our family who loved him dearly.

We are grateful.

— Vickie Carpenter

Bibliography

Chapter 2 — The Grass Juice Factor: A Discovery Ahead of Its Time

Cannon MD, Emerson GA (1939) Dietary Requirements of the Guinea Pig with Reference to the Need for a Special Factor. J Nutr 18:155–167. http://jn.nutrition.org/cgi/content/abstract/18/2/155

Kohler GO, Elvehjem CA, Hart EB (1938) The Relation of the "Grass Juice Factor" to Guinea Pig Nutrition. J Nutr 15:445–459. https://jn.nutrition.org/article/S0022-3166(23)12962-2/abstract

Kohler GO, Elvehjem CA, Hart EB (1939) The Relation of Pyrrole-Containing Pigments to Hemoglobin Synthesis. Journal of Biological Chemistry 128:501–509. https://linkinghub.elsevier.com/retrieve/pii/S0021925818737058

Randle SB, Sober HA, Kohler GO (1940) The Distribution of the "Grass Juice Factor" in Plant and Animal Materials. J Nutr 20:459–466. http://jn.nutrition.org/cgi/content/abstract/20/5/459

Connor Johnson B, Elvehjem CA, Peterson WH (1941) The Content of Grass-Juice Factor in Legume Silages and in Milk Produced Therefrom. J Dairy Sci 24:861–864. http://jds.fass.org/cgi/content/abstract/24/10/861

Mannering GJ, Cannon MD, Barki HV, Elvehjem CA, Hart EB (1943) Further Evidence for the Existence of Specific Dietary Essentials for the Guinea Pig. Journal of Biological Chemistry 151:101–107. http://www.sciencedirect.com/science/article/pii/S0021925818721170

Kohler GO (1944) The Effect of Stage of Growth on the Chemistry of the Grasses. Journal of Biological Chemistry 152:215–223. https://linkinghub.elsevier.com/retrieve/pii/S0021925818720449

Lakhanpal RK, Davis JR, Typpo JT, Briggs GM (1966) Evidence for an Unidentified Growth Factor(s) from Alfalfa and Other Plant Sources for Young Guinea Pigs. J Nutr 89:341–346. https://jn.nutrition.org/article/S0022-3166(23)14858-9/abstract

Singh KD, Morris ER, Regan WO, O'Dell BL (1968) An Unrecognized Nutrient for the Guinea Pig. J Nutr 94:534–542. https://jn.nutrition.org/article/S0022-3166(23)04948-9/abstract

Chapter 3 — Identifying the Grass Juice Factor

Osawa T, Katsuzaki H, Hagiwara Y, Hagiwara H, Shibamoto T (1992) A Novel Antioxidant Isolated from Young Green Barley Leaves. J Agric Food Chem 40:1135–1138. http://dx.doi.org/10.1021/jf00019a009

Markham KR, Mitchell KA (2003) The Mis-identification of the Major Antioxidant Flavonoids in Young Barley (Hordeum vulgare) Leaves. Z Naturforsch C J Biosci 58:53–56. http://www.ncbi.nlm.nih.gov/pubmed/12622226

Mohamed SM, Abdel-Rahim EA, Aly TA, Naguib AM, Khattab MS (2022) Barley Microgreen Incorporation in Diet-Controlled Diabetes and Counteracted Aflatoxicosis in Rats. Exp Biol Med (Maywood) 247:385–394. *(online 2021, in print 2022)* https://www.ncbi.nlm.nih.gov/pmc/articles/PMC8919319/

Chapter 4 — What Makes Barley Grass Juice Unique: Enzymes, Synergy, and the Living System

Seibold RL. Cereal Grass: Nature's Greatest Gift. Wilderness Community Education Foundation, 1991, pp. 12–18.

Chapter 5 — Metabolic Health and Diabetes

Mohamed RS, Marrez DA, Salem SH, Zaghloul AH, Ashoush IS, et al (2019) Hypoglycemic, Hypolipidemic and Antioxidant Effects of Green Sprouts Juice and Functional Dairy Micronutrients Against Streptozotocin-Induced Oxidative Stress and Diabetes in Rats. Heliyon 5. https://www.cell.com/heliyon/abstract/S2405-8440(18)38127-1

Mohamed SM, Abdel-Rahim EA, Aly TA, Naguib AM, Khattab MS (2022) Barley Microgreen Incorporation in Diet-Controlled Diabetes and Counteracted Aflatoxicosis in Rats. Exp Biol Med (Maywood) 247:385–394. *(same as reference 12)* https://www.ncbi.nlm.nih.gov/pmc/articles/PMC8919319/

Thatiparthi J, Dodoala S, Koganti B, Kvsrg P (2019) Barley Grass Juice (Hordeum vulgare L.) Inhibits Obesity and Improves Lipid Profile in High Fat Diet-Induced Rat Model. J Ethnopharmacol 238:111843. http://www.ncbi.nlm.nih.gov/pubmed/30951844

Khattab MS, Aly TAA, Mohamed SM, Naguib AMM, AL-Farga A, et al (2022) Hordeum vulgare L. Microgreen Mitigates Reproductive Dysfunction and Oxidative Stress in Streptozotocin-Induced Diabetes and Aflatoxicosis in Male Rats. Food Sci Nutr 10:3355–3367. https://www.ncbi.nlm.nih.gov/pmc/articles/PMC9548372/

Chapter 6 — Mental Health, Fatigue, and Stress

Shrivastava AK, Magar PT, Shrestha L (2022) Effect of Aqueous Extract of Barley and Wheat Grass in Stress Induced Depression in Swiss Mice. J Ayurveda Integr Med 13:100630. https://www.ncbi.nlm.nih.gov/pmc/articles/PMC9468397/

Yamaura K, Nakayama N, Shimada M, Bi Y, Fukata H, et al (2012) Antidepressant-Like Effects of Young Green Barley Leaf (Hordeum vulgare L.) in the Mouse Forced Swimming Test. Pharmacognosy Res 4:22–26. https://www.ncbi.nlm.nih.gov/pmc/articles/PMC3250035/

Yamaura K, Tanaka R, Bi Y, Fukata H, Oishi N, et al (2015) Protective Effect of Young Green Barley Leaf (Hordeum vulgare L.) on Restraint Stress-Induced Decrease in Hippocampal Brain-Derived Neurotrophic Factor in Mice. Pharmacogn Mag 11:S86–S92. https://www.ncbi.nlm.nih.gov/pmc/articles/PMC4461973/

Borah M, Sarma P, Das S (2014) A Study of the Protective Effect of *Triticum aestivum* L. in an Experimental Animal Model of Chronic Fatigue Syndrome. Pharmacognosy Res 6:285–291. https://www.ncbi.nlm.nih.gov/pmc/articles/PMC4166815/

Chapter 7 — Cancer Research and Cellular Protection

Czerwonka A, Kawka K, Cykier K, Lemieszek MK, Rzeski W (2017) Evaluation of Anticancer Activity of Water and Juice Extracts of Young Hordeum vulgare in Human Cancer Cell Lines HT-29 and A549. Ann Agric Environ Med 24:345–349. http://www.ncbi.nlm.nih.gov/pubmed/28664721

Kawka K, Lemieszek MK, Rzeski W (2019) Chemopreventive Properties of Young Green Barley Extracts in In Vitro Model of Colon Cancer. Ann Agric Environ Med 26:174–181. http://www.ncbi.nlm.nih.gov/pubmed/30922050

Lemieszek MK, Rzeski W (2020) Enhancement of Chemopreventive Properties of Young Green Barley and Chlorella Extracts Used Together Against Colon Cancer Cells. Ann Agric Environ Med 27:591–598. http://www.ncbi.nlm.nih.gov/pubmed/33356066

Lemieszek MK, Komaniecka I, Chojnacki M, Choma A, Rzeski W (2022) Immunomodulatory Properties of Polysaccharide-Rich Young Green Barley (Hordeum vulgare) Extract and Its Structural Characterization. Molecules 27:1742. https://www.ncbi.nlm.nih.gov/pmc/articles/PMC8911554/

Lemieszek MK, Rzeski W (2023) Synergism of Antiproliferative Effects of Young Green Barley and Chlorella Water Extracts Against Human Breast Cancer Cells. Ann Agric Environ Med 30:273–280. http://www.ncbi.nlm.nih.gov/pubmed/37387377

Li J, Zhang W, Xu H, Zhou L, Guo H, et al (2023) Barley Grass Juice Attenuates Hydrodynamic Transfection-Induced HCC Initiation in Mice. Nutr Cancer 75:750–760. http://www.ncbi.nlm.nih.gov/pubmed/36495148

Kubatka P, Kello M, Kajo K, Kruzliak P, Výbohová D, et al (2016) Young Barley Indicates Antitumor Effects in Experimental Breast Cancer In Vivo and In Vitro. Nutr Cancer 68:611–621. http://www.ncbi.nlm.nih.gov/pubmed/27042893

Yu D (2009) Laboratory Report on the Effect of BarleyMax on H2O2-Induced DNA Damage in HT29 Cells in the Comet Assay. Project Number BarleyMax2009-01. Cancer Chemoprotection Core Laboratory, Linus Pauling Institute, Oregon State University. Unpublished report commissioned by Hallelujah Acres.

Chapter 8 — Inflammation, Autoimmune Conditions, and Tissue Repair

Choi K-C, Hwang J-M, Bang S-J, Son Y-O, Kim B-T, et al (2013) Methanol Extract of the Aerial Parts of Barley (Hordeum vulgare) Suppresses Lipopolysaccharide-Induced Inflammatory Responses In Vitro and In Vivo. Pharm Biol 51:1066–1076. http://www.ncbi.nlm.nih.gov/pubmed/23746221

Kamiyama M, Shibamoto T (2012) Flavonoids with Potent Antioxidant Activity Found in Young Green Barley Leaves. J Agric Food Chem 60:6260–6267. http://dx.doi.org/10.1021/jf301700j

Seo KH, Park MJ, Ra J-E, Han S-I, Nam M-H, Kim JH, Lee JH, Seo WD (2014) Saponarin from Barley Sprouts Inhibits NF-κB and MAPK on LPS-Induced RAW 264.7 Cells. *Food Funct* 5:3005–3013. https://pubmed.ncbi.nlm.nih.gov/25238253/

Yang JY, Woo S-Y, Lee MJ, Kim HY, Lee JH, Kim S-H, Seo WD (2021) Lutonarin from Barley Seedlings Inhibits the Lipopolysaccharide-Stimulated Inflammatory

Response of RAW 264.7 Macrophages by Suppressing Nuclear Factor-κB Signaling. *Molecules* 26:1571. https://www.mdpi.com/1420-3049/26/6/1571

Cremer L, Herold A, Avram D, Szegli G (1998) A Purified Green Barley Extract with Modulatory Properties upon TNF Alpha and ROS Released by Human Specialised Cells Isolated from RA Patients. Roum Arch Microbiol Immunol 57:231–242. https://pubmed.ncbi.nlm.nih.gov/11845435/

Feng Y, Li D, Ma C, Tian M, Hu X, Chen F (2022) Barley Leaf Ameliorates *Citrobacter rodentium*-Induced Colitis through Preventive Effects. Nutrients 14:3833. https://pmc.ncbi.nlm.nih.gov/articles/PMC9502111/

Ben-Arye E, Goldin E, Wengrower D, Stamper A, Kohn R, et al (2002) Wheat Grass Juice in the Treatment of Active Distal Ulcerative Colitis: A Randomized Double-Blind Placebo-Controlled Trial. Scand J Gastroenterol 37:444–449. http://www.ncbi.nlm.nih.gov/pubmed/11989836

Nepali S, Ki H-H, Lee J-H, Lee H-Y, Kim D-K, et al (2017) Wheatgrass-Derived Polysaccharide Has Antiinflammatory, Anti-Oxidative and Anti-Apoptotic Effects on LPS-Induced Hepatic Injury in Mice. Phytother Res 31:1107–1116. http://www.ncbi.nlm.nih.gov/pubmed/28543910

Panthi M, Subba RK, Raut B, Khanal DP, Koirala N (2020) Bioactivity Evaluations of Leaf Extract Fractions from Young Barley Grass and Correlation with Their Phytochemical Profiles. BMC Complement Med Ther 20:64. https://www.ncbi.nlm.nih.gov/pmc/articles/PMC7076879/

Karbarz M, Mytych J, Solek P, Stawarczyk K, Tabecka-Lonczynska A, et al (2019) Cereal Grass Juice in Wound Healing: Hormesis and Cell-Survival in Normal Fibroblasts, in Contrast to Toxic Events in Cancer Cells. J Physiol Pharmacol 70. http://www.ncbi.nlm.nih.gov/pubmed/31741456

Chapter 10 — Enzymes, Chlorophyll, and the Water Test

López-Ayerra B, Murcia MA, Garcia-Carmona F (1998) Lipid Peroxidation and Chlorophyll Levels in Spinach During Refrigerated Storage and After Industrial Processing. Food Chemistry 61:113–118. https://www.sciencedirect.com/science/article/pii/S030881469700099X

Donaldson MS (2003) Unpublished Analysis of Chlorophyll Degradation in Barley Grass Products. Hallelujah Acres Raw Food Lab.

About the Author

Michael Donaldson, PhD, is a chemical engineer and independent nutrition researcher with more than 28 years of experience in raw food science. He holds a doctorate in chemical engineering from Cornell University, with an emphasis in biochemical engineering.

After completing his graduate studies, Dr. Donaldson joined Hallelujah Diet, where he became the organization's one-man research department, developing enzyme-based analytical methods to evaluate the biological vitality of raw food products. That work grew out of a deceptively simple question: how do you prove, scientifically, that a food has not been cooked? The methodology he developed became the foundation for more than two decades of independent comparative testing of barley grass juice powders and other green food products available in the United States market.

His research has spanned a wide range of nutrition topics — including dietary interventions, bone health, metabolic disease, and micronutrient science — with a particular focus on the intersection of analytical chemistry and whole-food nutrition: understanding not just what living foods contain, but whether what they contain survives the journey from field to consumer. He lives in Zillah, Washington. Learn more about his research at twhealthprod-ucts.com.

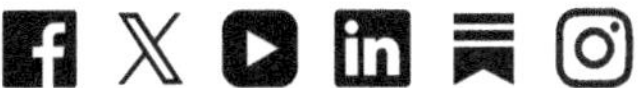

www.ingramcontent.com/pod-product-compliance
Lightning Source LLC
Chambersburg PA
CBHW071349150726
47997CB00002B/907